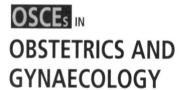

OSCEs IN
OBSTETRICS AND
GYNAECOLOGY

To Roger and Ammy, our support systems

For Churchill Livingstone:

Publisher: Timothy Horne
Project Manager: Ninette Premdas
Project Editor: Jim Killgore
Design Direction: Erik Bigland
Project Controller: Nancy Arnott

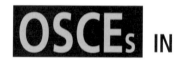

OSCEs IN
OBSTETRICS AND GYNAECOLOGY

JANICE RYMER MD MRCOG FRNZCOG

Senior Lecturer/Consultant in Obstetrics and Gynaecology,
UMDS, Guy's and St. Thomas' Hospitals Trust, London, UK

HASIB AHMED MRCOG

Consultant in Obstetrics and Gynaecology,
Medway Hospital Trust, Kent, UK

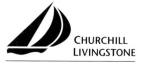

**CHURCHILL
LIVINGSTONE**

EDINBURGH LONDON NEW YORK PHILADELPHIA SYDNEY
TORONTO 1998

CHURCHILL LIVINGSTONE
An imprint of Harcourt Publishers Limited

© Churchill Livingstone, a division of Harcourt Brace & Company Limited 1998
© Harcourt Publishers Limited 1999

◢▶ is a registered trademark of Harcourt Publishers Limited.

J Rymer and H Ahmed have asserted their rights under the Copyright, Design and
Patents Act, 1988, to be identified as Authors of this work.

First Edition 1998
  Reprinted 1999

0443-05610-2

British Library Cataloguing in Publication Data
A catalogue record for this book is available from the British Library

Library of Congress Cataloging in Publication Data
A catalog record for this book is available from the Library of Congress

Medical Knowledge is constantly changing. As new information becomes available,
changes in treatment procedures, equipment and the use of drugs become necessary.
The authors and publisher have, as far as it is possible, taken care to ensure that the
information given in this text is accurate and up to date. However, readers are strongly
advised to confirm that the information, especially with regard to drug usage, complies
with current legislation and standards of practice.

The
publisher's
policy is to use
**paper manufactured
from sustainable forests**

Produced by Addison Wesley Longman China Limited, Hong Kong
SWTC/02

PREFACE

This textbook on the Objective Structured Clinical Examinations (OSCEs) in Obstetrics and Gynaecology aims to give the undergraduate and postgraduate extensive coverage of topics in obstetrics, gynaecology, contraception, neonatal medicine and sexually transmitted diseases. We have ensured that there is a good mix of topics within each circuit of the OSCE, therefore providing the student with opportunities for comprehensive revision. We have organized the structured oral and communication stations into a separate section, as this is more appropriate in a non-interactive format.

It is not possible to produce a book like this without the help of colleagues and friends and we would particularly like to thank Mr. Alfred Cutner, Consultant Gynaecologist, and the Photographic Departments of Guy's Hospital and Medway Trust Hospital. We are also eternally grateful to the patients of Guy's Hospital and Medway Trust Hospital for volunteering themselves to be photographed. We sought the advice both of a general practitioner and of a research Fellow at the cutting edge of obstetrics and gynaecology and are grateful to Dr. Joe Rosenthal, Senior Lecturer in General Practice at the Royal Free Hospital, and Mr Edward Morris, Research Fellow in Gynaecology at Guy's Hospital, for reviewing the book and advising us on the questions. Finally, we would like to thank Tracy Alderton who has typed the manuscript tirelessly and with never-ending cheerfulness. We hope that this book will be invaluable for both undergraduate and postgraduate preparation for OSCEs in obstetrics and gynaecology.

London
1998

J. R.
H. A.

CONTENTS

INTRODUCTION TO OSCEs

Objective structured clinical examinations (OSCEs) as a method of student assessment are well established and are gradually being introduced into postgraduate assessment. OSCEs have been developed because they are valid, reliable, have high fidelity and are a feasible method of assessment.

Depending on the particular examination there are a varying number of stations. At each station the candidate has to perform a task, and these stations may be testing knowledge, skills, communication or problem-solving ability. Depending on the type of station, there may be a role player, a patient, a photograph, a pelvic model or a clinical scenario.

At each station you have a defined period of time at the end of which a bell or buzzer sounds and you move on, usually in a clockwise direction, to the next station. Within the OSCE circuit there may be rest stations and these stations often provide information to prepare you for the following station.

Within this book we have arranged four typical OSCE circuits. Each of these circuits consists of 20 stations. As it is impossible to be interactive in a book, we have organised the structured orals and communication stations separately. Normally within an OSCE circuit the interactive and the structured oral stations would be intermingled with the other stations.

Knowledge or factual stations
These stations are purely assessing your knowledge regarding certain subjects. The material provided may be a photograph, results of investigations or a clinical scenario. Within the four following circuits there are many examples of these. When performing an OSCE, be certain to listen carefully to the examiner's instructions as to where to write on your answer sheet.

Clinical skills stations
At these stations there may well be patients on whom you are asked to perform a skill. With regard to pelvic examinations, it is unlikely that there will be live patients and more commonly you would be asked to do a speculum examination or bimanual examination on a plastic model. If you are put into the situation of examining a plastic model, it would be appropriate to talk to the model as if it were a live patient to show that you are quite accustomed to this scenario.

Summary
An OSCE ensures that each candidate is exposed to the same examination questions and environment. Therefore the marking is very rigid and standardized.

CIRCUIT A

1.1 Look at the photograph and state three differential diagnoses.

1.2 What three symptoms may she have presented with?

1.3 Name three appropriate investigations.

1.4 What corrective procedure should she have?

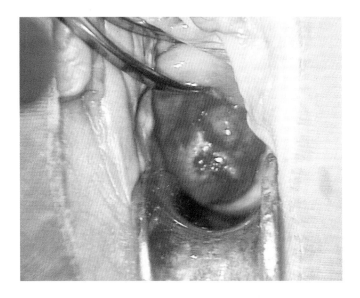

2.1   The baby in the photograph is 2 days old. What treatment is he receiving?

2.2   Name the condition that is being treated.

2.3   In this case the cause was physiological. Describe the mechanisms of jaundice. Specify three points.

2.4   How is unconjugated bilirubin transported in the serum?

2.5   Describe two clinical features of kernicterus other than jaundice.

2.6   Name two potential long-term sequelae of kernicterus.

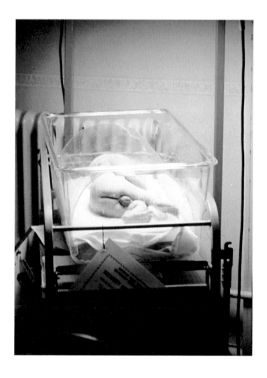

3.1 What are these pills used for?

3.2 What do these pills (excluding the larger pills) contain?

3.3 Apart from the obvious benefit of this medication, name four other benefits.

3.4 If a woman missed the last two pills in the red section, what would you advise her to do?

3.5 Name two absolute contraindications to this preparation.

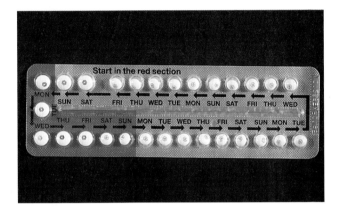

A woman (para 2 gravida 3) presented at 33 weeks with vaginal bleeding. Her ultrasound scan (USS) is illustrated. (Her first delivery was by lower segment caesarean section (LSCS), and her second was a normal delivery.) Her blood group is O rhesus positive.

4.1 What is the cause of her bleeding?

4.2 What would you have found on abdominal examination? Name two features.

4.3 What would your management of this woman be? Name two aspects.

4.4 How would you deliver her?

4.5 If the placenta was anterior, would anything concern you?

4.6 Name three other causes of antepartum haemorrhage (APH) at 33 weeks.

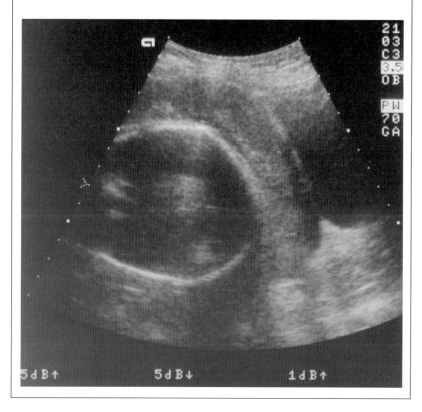

Mrs MK has had a bivalent screening test performed in this pregnancy. The result is shown.

5.1 Which two parameters have been measured?

5.2 Which third parameter is usually measured in a trivalent test?

5.3 In the results, what does MOM stand for?

5.4 In this case, screening was performed because of raised maternal age. What is the risk of Down's syndrome in this pregnancy based on maternal age alone?

5.5 What is the risk of Down's syndrome based on the results of the bivalent test?

5.6 Comment on the significance of this result.

5.7 What is the risk of neural tube defect (NTD) in this woman?

5.8 Name two diagnostic tests which may be appropriate for Mrs MK.

Prenatal Maternal Serum Screening Report   **Report Date: 23-04-96**

Report Address   **Patient Information**
Mr H   Name   : K , M
Antenatal Clinic   Hospital Number : 571101
All Saints Hospital   Sample Number   : 109646
Magpie Hall Road   Specimen   First
Chatham ME4 5NG

Clinical Data

Date of Birth	: 01-11-57	LMP	: 20-12-95
Date Collected	: 15-04-96	Previous NTD	: None
Maternal Age at EDC	: 38	Previous Down's	: None
Maternal Weight	: 132.0 Kgs	Ethnic Group	: Caucasian
Multiple Pregnancy	: No	IDDM	: No

Screening Determinations

Gestational Age   : 17 weeks 1 days (by sonar)
MS-AFP Level   : 12.0   KU/L   ;   0.56 MoM
MS-Free-Beta Level   : 17.3   IU/L   ;   2.99 MoM

ONTD Interpretation : **Normal**
Comment   : This patient's AFP level is within normative range for the given gestational age.

ONTD Risks   : Open spina bifida   1 in >10,000
                       Anencephaly   1 in >10,000

Down's Interpretation : **Still At Risk**
Comment   : Down's risk is greater than the cut-off. However, age-related risk is also greater than the cut-off.

Risk of Down's   : 1 in 25 (At term)
Prior Risk of Down's : 1 in 189, based on maternal age only.

A 24-year-old primigravida presents at 32 weeks with a history of a large loss of clear fluid from the vagina.

6.1 How would you confirm the diagnosis of premature rupture of membranes (PROM)?

6.2 What is the differential diagnosis? Name two conditions.

6.3 What investigations would you perform? Name three.

6.4 What drug treatment might you consider and why? Name three drugs.

6.5 What is the percentage chance of spontaneous labour within the next 10 days?

A woman presents to the gynaecology clinic with an offensive vaginal discharge. The speculum examination shown below is performed.

7.1 Describe what you see.

7.2 You take a high vaginal sample, mix it with a drop of saline and look at it under the microscope. You see a flagellate parasite. What is the diagnosis?

7.3 Where else (apart from the vagina) would you find this organism?

7.4 How is this organism acquired?

7.5 What other organism is often found in association with it?

7.6 Name three aspects of your management.

7.7 What follow-up would you arrange?

7.8 What is the commonest cause of vaginal discharge?

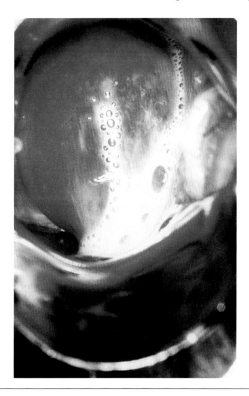

8.1 What abnormality do you see in the illustration?

8.2 What is the 'group' of abnormalities called?

8.3 What other group of abnormalities would this alert you to?

8.4 What symptoms may this woman present with? Name two.

8.5 If this woman were to become pregnant, what problems may she encounter in labour? Name two.

8.6 Name two structures of which the paramesonephic ducts are precursors?

8.7 What does the lower third of the vagina develop from?

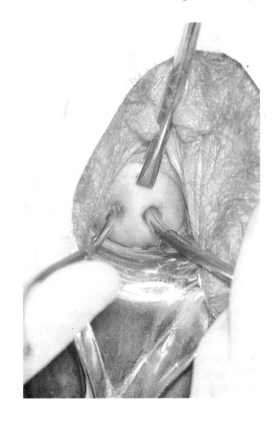

Look at the photograph.

9.1 Regarding the report shown, name the three major classification groups of maternal deaths.

9.2 In the report, what were the three commonest causes for direct maternal deaths (in the correct order)?

9.3 In a pregnant woman with a history of previous deep vein thrombosis in pregnancy, what are the RCOG recommendations for treatment? State medication, when to start and duration of therapy.

9.4 In a higher risk woman (multiple thromboembolic events in pregnancy), what are the recommendations?

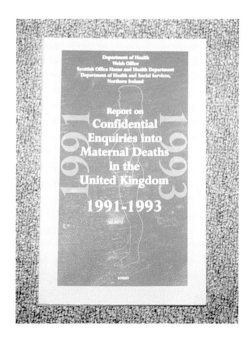

A 38-year-old primigravid woman has been admitted at 33 weeks gestation. She booked with a blood pressure (BP) of 110/60 mmHg. She has 2+ proteinuria and her BP is consistently 175/105 mmHg. She is complaining of visual disturbances.

10.1 What abnormalities are revealed in the haematology result? Name two.

10.2 Name two further maternal investigations you would arrange.

10.3 Name three principal risks for the woman and her fetus that would concern you.

10.4 She develops abdominal pain. What are the two most likely causes?

10.5 Her BP that afternoon goes up to 175/110. What antihypertensive would you give her in the first instance (and state the correct dose)?

Guy's Hospital **Department of Haematology**		Surname	A
		Forename	F
Date 10.9.97		Sex	F
		DOB	30.9.60
		Number	660435
Haemoglobin	13.4 g/dl		
White Cell Count	$9.3 \times 10^9/l$		
Platelet Count	$94 \times 10^{12}/l$		
PCV	0.45		
MCV	83 fl		
MCHC	29 g/dl		

Miss SE is 19 years old and is in her first pregnancy. Her last menstrual period was approximately 2 months ago and was normal. Her GP has carried out a pregnancy test, which was positive and has sent her for a transvaginal ultrasound scan. He is concerned because Miss SE has been complaining of pain and tenderness in the right iliac fossa. A photograph of the ultrasound findings is shown.

11.1 Describe the appearance of the uterine cavity. Name two features.

11.2 What organs giving rise to A and B are seen adjacent to the uterus?

11.3 What must be visualised during real-time ultrasound scanning to confirm that the fetus is alive?

11.4 What is the likely aetiology of B?

11.5 What is the usual outcome of B?

11.6 What two complications may occur with B and result in abdominal pain?

11.7 What is the function of B?

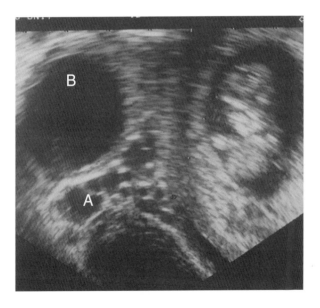

Mrs PP gave birth to a live baby boy 2 weeks ago. The midwife looking after her is worried because Mrs PP is not showing much interest in her newborn son. She spends a lot of the day in bed and is tearful.

12.1 What is the likely diagnosis?

12.2 Name three features which would confirm your diagnosis.

12.3 How common is the problem?

12.4 List three risk factors for postnatal depression.

12.5 Name two types of drugs that may be prescribed for Mrs PP.

13.1 Name the four hormones.

13.2 What two types of cells are involved in the synthesis of C?

13.3 What cells produce D?

13.4 What effect does D have on cervical mucus?

13.5 What hormone causes the temperature rise illustrated?

13.6 At birth, how many oocytes are present?

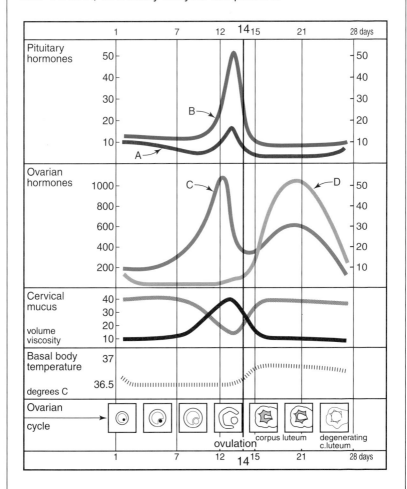

A 30-year-old, para 2 gravida 2 woman presents to the gynaecology clinic saying that she has premenstrual syndrome (PMS).

14.1 What is the commonest reported psychological symptom of PMS?

14.2 What are the two most common physical symptoms of PMS?

14.3 How do you make the diagnosis?

14.4 What relieves PMS physiologically?

14.5 Name five treatments.

The illustrated USS is from a 74-year-old woman.

15.1 Describe the scan. Name three features.

15.2 What is the most likely diagnosis?

15.3 What operation would be performed?

15.4 Name two symptoms she may have presented with.

15.5 What three methods may be used to screen for this disease?

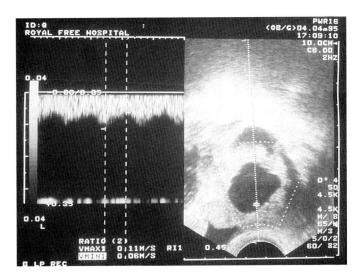

This 74-year-old presented with a 'lump' down below.

16.1 What is the diagnosis?

16.2 What is the main predisposing factor?

16.3 What conservative therapy could be instituted?

16.4 What surgical therapy could be offered?

16.5 Why might this present postmenopausally?

16.6 If she presented 2 years later with vault prolapse, what surgical operations could you offer? Name two.

16.7 In the outpatient department, what instrument would you use to examine this woman?

16.8 Name two conditions that may aggravate this condition?

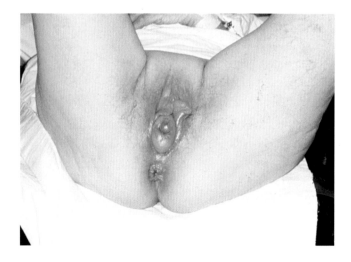

17.1 What two abnormalities does the X-ray show?

17.2 Name three symptoms she may have.

17.3 What other investigations would you order? Name three.

17.4 What is the probable diagnosis?

17.5 Name one treatment.

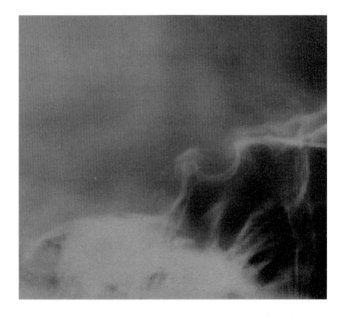

18.1 Name the three types of breech illustrated.

18.2 Name two maternal causes.

18.3 Name two fetal causes.

18.4 What two investigations would you perform in a primigravida at 37 weeks with a breech presentation if you were contemplating a vaginal delivery?

18.5 At term, what is the incidence of breech presentation?

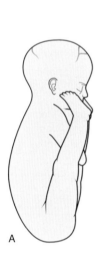

A

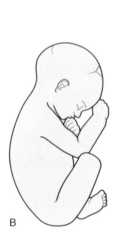

B

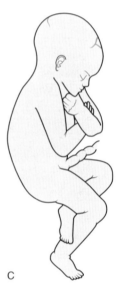

C

Mrs MR is 39 years old and has two children aged 14 and 11 who are alive and well. She is now 18 weeks pregnant and had an amniocentesis 2 weeks ago. The result is shown.

19.1 What is the risk of miscarriage associated with an amniocentesis procedure?

19.2 List four other complications that have been described following amniocentesis.

19.3 What is an alternative procedure to amniocentesis which yields a quicker cell culture for karyotyping?

19.4 After explaining the result to Mrs MR, what intervention should be discussed?

19.5 List three medical methods which may be used to perform this intervention.

Guy's Hospital **Department of Cytogenetics**	Surname	R
	Forename	M
Date 8.3.97	Sex	F
	DOB	22.10.58
	Number	S70719

Karyotype Report

Sample	Amniotic fluid
Cell culture	+ve
Karyotype	47 XY
Male fetus with trisomy 21	

Suggest review by Obstetrician ASAP

A measurement is being performed on the woman shown below.

20.1 What are the causes of large for dates? Name five.

20.2 Name three investigations you would perform.

20.3 What is the measurement called?

20.4 What is its relevance?

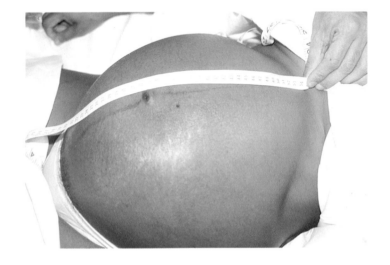

1.1 Look at the photograph and state three differential diagnoses. [Marks 3]
1. **Cervical carcinoma**
2. **Cervical polyp**
3. **Endometrial polyp/fibroid polyp**

1.2 What three symptoms may she have presented with? [Marks 3]
1. **Postcoital bleeding**
2. **Intermenstrual bleeding**
3. **Menorrhagia**

1.3 Name three appropriate investigations. [Marks 3]
1. **TVS**
2. **Cervical smear**
3. **Endometrial biopsy**
4. **Hysteroscopy**
5. **Biopsy of lesion**

1.4 What corrective procedure should she have? [Marks 1]
1. **Removal of polyp**
2. **Excision biopsy of lesion**

2.1 The baby in the photograph is 2 days old. What treatment is he receiving? [Marks 1]
Phototherapy

2.2 Name the condition that is being treated. [Marks 1]
Jaundice (raised serum bilirubin)

2.3 In this case the cause was physiological. Describe the mechanisms of jaundice. (Specify three points.) [Marks 3]
1. **Raised neonatal PCV**
2. **Immature liver**
3. **Poor conjugation**
4. **Dehydration**
5. **Raised unconjugated bilirubin**

2.4 How is unconjugated bilirubin transported in the serum?
[Marks 1]
Bound to albumin

2.5 Describe two clinical features of kernicterus other than jaundice. [Marks 2]
1. **Poor feeding**
2. **Drowsiness**
3. **Opisthotonos**
4. **Convulsions**

2.6 Name two potential long-term sequelae of kernicterus.
[Marks 2]
1. **Residual brain damage**
2. **Choreoathetosis**
3. **Mental retardation**

STATION 3	ANSWERS	CIRCUIT A

3.1 What are these pills used for? [Marks 1]
Contraception

3.2 What do these pills (excluding the larger pills) contain?
[Marks 2]
1. **Oestrogen**
2. **Progestogen**

3.3 Apart from the obvious benefit of this medication, name four other benefits. [Marks 4]
1. **Cycle control**
2. **Less bleeding**
3. **Less pain**
4. **Protects against ovarian cancer**
5. **Protects against endometrial cancer**
6. **Prevents bone loss**
7. **Alleviates symptoms of endometriosis**
8. **Acne improvement**
9. **Protects against PID**

3.4 If a woman missed the last two pills in the red section, what would you advise her to do? [Marks 1]
Nothing

3.5 Name two absolute contraindications to this preparation. [Marks 2]
1. **Past history of DVT**
2. **Past history of CVA**
3. **Focal migraine**
4. **Gross obesity**
5. **>40 cigarettes/day**
6. **High blood pressure**
7. **Severe diabetes**

STATION 4	ANSWERS	CIRCUIT A

4.1 What is the cause of her bleeding? [Marks 1]
Placenta praevia

4.2 What would you have found on abdominal examination? Name two features. [Marks 2]
1. **Soft uterus**
2. **Presenting part high**

4.3 What would your management of this woman be? Name two aspects. [Marks 2]
1. **Keep in hospital**
2. **Always have blood available/Group and cross-match**
3. **IV (intravenous) line**

4.4 How would you deliver her? [Marks 1]
LSCS

4.5 If the placenta was anterior, would anything concern you? [Marks 1]
The possibility of morbid adherence of the placenta

4.6 Name three other causes of APH at 33 weeks. [Marks 3]
1. **Abruption**
2. **Marginal edge bleed**
3. **Vasa praevia**
4. **Local causes**

STATION 5	ANSWERS	CIRCUIT A

5.1 Which two parameters have been measured? [Marks 2]
1. **Serum alpha-feto-protein**
2. **Serum beta human chorionic gonadotrophin**

5.2 Which third parameter is usually measured in a trivalent test? [Marks 1]
Serum oestriol

5.3 In the results, what does MOM stand for? [Marks 1]
Multiples of the median

5.4 In this case, screening was performed because of raised maternal age. What is the risk of Down's syndrome in this pregnancy based on maternal age alone? [Marks 1]
1:189

5.5 What is the risk of Down's syndrome based on the results of the bivalent test? [Marks 1]
1:25

5.6 Comment on the significance of this result. [Marks 1]
There is a higher risk of Down's based on the result compared with that based on age alone, i.e. a positive screening result.

5.7 What is the risk of NTD in this woman? [Marks 1]
1 in >10000

5.8 Name two diagnostic tests which may be appropriate for Mrs MK. [Marks 2]
   1. Amniocentesis
   2. Chorion villus biopsy/placental biopsy
   3. Fetal blood sampling

STATION 6	ANSWERS	CIRCUIT A

6.1 How would you confirm the diagnosis of PROM? [Marks 1]
Speculum examination and see pooling of liquor in the vagina

6.2 What is the differential diagnosis? Name two conditions. [Marks 2]
   1. Urinary incontinence
   2. Vaginal discharge

6.3 What investigations would you perform? Name three. [Marks 3]
1. **Endocervical swab**
2. **White blood count (WBC)**
3. **Ultrasound scan**
4. **Fibronectin swab**
5. **C-reactive (CR) protein**
6. **Mid-stream urine (MSU)**

6.4 What drug treatment might you consider and why? Name three drugs. [Marks 3]
1. **Tocolysis if contracting**
2. **Steroids for lung maturation**
3. **Antibiotics for prophylaxis**

6.5 What is the percentage chance of spontaneous labour within the next 10 days? [Marks 1]
>90%

STATION 7	ANSWERS	CIRCUIT A

7.1 Describe what you see. [Marks 1]
A frothy yellowy white discharge

7.2 You take a high vaginal sample, mix it with a drop of saline and look at it under the microscope. You see a flagellate parasite. What is the diagnosis? [Marks 1]
Trichomonas vaginalis

7.3 Where else (apart from the vagina) would you find this organism? [Marks 1]
1. **Uretha**
2. **Upper genital tract/endocervix**

7.4 How is this organism acquired? [Marks 1]
Sexually

7.5 What other organism is often found in association with it? [Marks 1]
Gonococcus

7.6 Name three aspects of your management. [Marks 3]
1. **Metronidazole**

2. Screen for other sexually transmitted diseases
3. Advise barrier contraception until disease resolves
4. Screen and treat the partner/partners

7.7 What follow-up would you arrange? [Marks 1]
Repeat swabs after treatment

7.8 What is the commonest cause of vaginal discharge? [Marks 1]
Candida

STATION 8	ANSWERS	CIRCUIT A

8.1 What abnormality do you see in the illustration? [Marks 1]
Two cervices

8.2 What is the 'group' of abnormalities called? [Marks 1]
Müllerian duct abnormalities

8.3 What other group of abnormalities would this alert you do? [Marks 1]
Renal tract abnormalities

8.4 What symptoms may this woman present with? Name two. [Marks 2]
1. **Recurrent miscarriage**
2. **Infertility**
3. **Menorrhagia**

8.5 If this woman were to become pregnant, what problems may she encounter in labour? Name two. [Marks 2]
1. **Incoordinate uterine action**
2. **Malpresentations**
3. **Retained placenta**

8.6 Name two structures of which the paramesonephic ducts are precursors? [Marks 2]
1. **Fallopian tubes**
2. **Uterus**
3. **Upper two-thirds of the vagina**

8.7 What does the lower third of the vagina develop from? [Marks 1]
Urogenital sinus

9.1 Regarding the report shown, name the three major classification groups of maternal deaths. [Marks 3]
1. **Direct**
2. **Indirect**
3. **Fortuitous**

9.2 In the report, what were the three commonest causes for direct maternal deaths (in the correct order)? [Marks 3]
1. **Thrombosis/thromboembolism**
2. **Hypertensive disorders of pregnancy**
3. **Haemorrhage**

9.3 In a pregnant woman with a history of previous deep vein thrombosis in pregnancy, what are the RCOG recommendations for treatment? State medication, when to start and duration of therapy. [Marks 3]
1. **Heparin (with or without warfarin)**
2. **Start after delivery**
3. **Continue for up to 6 weeks**

9.4 In a higher risk woman (multiple thromboembolic events in pregnancy), what are the recommendations? [Marks 1]
Subcutaneous heparin throughout pregnancy

10.1 What abnormalities are revealed in the haematology result? Name two. [Marks 2]
1. **Haemoconcentration/high haemoglobin/high packed cell volume (PCV)**
2. **Low platelets**

10.2 Name two further maternal investigations you would arrange. [Marks 2]
1. **24 hour urinalysis for protein**
2. **Liver function tests**
3. **MSU**
4. **Clotting studies**
5. **Serum urea and electrolytes (U&E)**
6. **Urate**

10.3 Name three principal risks for the woman and her fetus that would concern you. [Marks 3]
1. **Eclampsia**

2. **Abruption causing fetal distress**
3. **Death**
4. **Disseminated intravascular coagulation (DIC)**
5. **Cerebrovascular accident**

10.4 She develops abdominal pain. What are the two most likely causes? [Marks 2]
1. **Liver tenderness – subcapsular haemorrhages**
2. **Placental abruption**

10.5 Her BP that afternoon goes up to 175/110. What antihypertensive would you give her in the first instance (and state the correct dose)? [Marks 1]
1. **Hydrallazine (initially in a 5 mg i.v. bolus)**
2. **Nifedipine (10 mg sublingually)**

STATION 11	ANSWERS	CIRCUIT A

11.1 Describe the appearance of the uterine cavity. Name two features. [Marks 2]
1. **Intrauterine gestation sac**
2. **Identifiable fetus within the gestation sac**

11.2 What organs giving rise to A and B are seen adjacent to the uterus? [Marks 2]
A – bowel
B – Ovary

11.3 What must be visualised during real-time ultrasound scanning to confirm that the fetus is alive? [Marks 1]
Fetal heart movement

11.4 What is the likely aetiology of B? [Marks 1]
Corpus luteum cyst of pregnancy

11.5 What is the usual outcome of B? [Marks 1]
Spontaneous resolution by the end of the first trimester

11.6 What two complications may occur with B and result in abdominal pain? [Marks 2]
1. **Cyst haemorrhage/(rupture)**
2. **Cyst/ovarian torsion**

11.7 What is the function of B? [Marks 1]
Steroid hormone secretion in first trimester/oestrogen progestogen secretion in first trimester.

12.1 What is the likely diagnosis? [Marks 1]
Postnatal depression

12.2 Name three features which would confirm your diagnosis. [Marks 3]
1. **Insomia**
2. **Loss of appetite**
3. **Irritability**
4. **Inability to cope**
5. **Self-reproach**

12.3 How common is the problem? [Marks 1]
Approximately 25% of new mothers (20%–30%)

12.4 List three risk factors for postnatal depression. [Marks 3]
1. **Depression in index pregnancy**
2. **Age >30**
3. **History of depression/previous postnatal depression**
4. **History of severe pre-menstrual syndrome**
5. **Poor socioeconomic support**
6. **Traumatic pregnancy/delivery**
7. **Poor neonatal outcome**

12.5 Name two types of drugs that may be prescribed for Mrs PP. [Marks 2]
1. **Oestrogens**
2. **Progestogens**
3. **Antidepressants**

13.1 Name the four hormones. [Marks 4]
A. **FSH**
B. **LH**
C. **Oestradiol**
D. **Progesterone**

13.2 What two types of cells are involved in the synthesis of C? [Marks 2]
1. **Theca cells of the stroma**
2. **Granulosa cells of the follicle**

13.3 What cells produce D? [Marks 1]
Luteinised granulosa cells of the corpus luteum

13.4 What effect does D have on cervical mucus? [Marks 1]
It makes mucus hostile or impenetrable to sperm

13.5 What hormone causes the temperature rise illustrated? [Marks 1]
Progesterone

13.6 At birth, how many oocytes are present? [Marks 1]
2 million (1–4 million)

STATION 14	ANSWERS	CIRCUIT A

14.1 What is the commonest reported psychological symptom of PMS? [Marks 1]
Irritability

14.2 What are the two most common physical symptoms of PMS? [Marks 2]
1. **Abdominal bloating**
2. **Breast tenderness**

14.3 How do you make the diagnosis? [Marks 1]
Menstrual symptom diary

14.4 What relieves PMS physiologically? [Marks 1]
Onset of menstruation

14.5 Name five treatments. [Marks 5]
1. **Explanation and reassurance**
2. **Relaxation techniques**
3. **Combined oral contraception (COC)/hormone replacement therapy (HRT)**
4. **Nonsteroidal anti-inflammatory drugs (NSAIDs)**
5. **Pyridoxine**
6. **Bromocriptine**
7. **Evening primrose oil**
8. **Diuretics**

STATION 15	ANSWERS	CIRCUIT A

15.1 Describe the scan. Name three features. [Marks 3]
1. **Cystic structure**
2. **Solid elements**
3. **Smooth capsule**
4. **Free fluid**

15.2 What is the most likely diagnosis? [Marks 1]
Ovarian carcinoma

15.3 What operation would be performed? [Marks 1]
1. **Staging laparotomy**
2. **TAH and BSO and omentectomy**

15.4 Name two symptoms she may have presented with. [Marks 2]
1. **Abdominal distention**
2. **Pressure effects on other organs**
3. **Problems in micturation/defaecation**
4. **Pelvic pain/abdominal pain**

15.5 What three methods may be used to screen for this disease? [Marks 3]
1. **Tumour markers**
2. **Vaginal ultrasound**
3. **Vaginal examination**
4. **Doppler bloodflow**

STATION 16 ANSWERS **CIRCUIT A**

16.1 What is the diagnosis? [Marks 1]
Uterovaginal prolapse/procidentia

16.2 What is the main predisposing factor? [Marks 1]
Childbirth

16.3 What conservative therapy could be instituted? [Marks 1]
Ring pessary/shelf pessary

16.4 What surgical therapy could be offered? [Marks 1]
Vaginal hysterectomy, anterior and posterior repair

16.5 Why might this present postmenopausally? [Marks 1]
Lack of oestrogen

16.6 If she presented 2 years later with vault prolapse, what surgical operations could you offer? Name two. [Marks 2]
1. **Le Forts procedure**
2. **Sacrospinous fixation**
3. **Sacrocolpopexy**
4. **Moscowitz procedure**

16.7 In the outpatient department what instrument would you use to examine this woman? [Marks 1]
Sim's speculum

16.8 Name two conditions that may aggravate this condition? [Marks 2]
1. **Chronic cough**
2. **Constipation**
3. **Pelvic mass**
4. **Obesity**

17.1 What two abnormalities does the X-ray show? [Marks 2]
1. **Double flooring of the pituitary fossa**
2. **Enlargement of the pituitary fossa**

17.2 Name three symptoms she may have. [Marks 3]
1. **Galactorrhoea**
2. **Amenorrhoea**
3. **Visual sypmtoms**
4. **Headaches**
5. **Infertility**

17.3 What other investigations would you order? Name three. [Marks 3]
1. **Serum prolactin**
2. **Visual fields mapping**
3. **Thyroid function tests**
4. **MRI/CT of the pituitary fossa**

17.4 What is the probable diagnosis? [Marks 1]
Pituitary adenoma

17.5 Name one treatment. [Marks 1]
1. **Bromocriptine/carbergoline**
2. **Hypophysectomy**
3. **Radiation therapy**

18.1 Name the three types of breech illustrated. [Marks 3]
A – extended/frank
B – flexed
C – footling

18.2 Name two maternal causes. [Marks 2]
   1. **Grand multiparity**
   2. **Uterine anomalies**
   3. **Pelvic tumour**
   4. **Bony pelvic abnormality**

18.3 Name two fetal causes. [Marks 2]
   1. **Fetal abnormality**
   2. **Extended neck**
   3. **Multiple gestation**
   4. **Prematurity**

18.4 What two investigations would you perform in a primigravida at 37 weeks with a breech presentation if you were contemplating a vaginal delivery? [Marks 2]
   1. **USS**
   2. **Erect lateral pelvimetry/CT pelvimetry**

18.5 At term, what is the incidence of breech presentation? [Marks 1]
   Less than 5%

19.1 What is the risk of miscarriage associated with an amniocentesis procedure? [Marks 1]
   1:100

19.2 List four other complications that have been described following amniocentesis. [Marks 4]
   1. **Oligohydramnios**
   2. **Amniotic bands**
   3. **Talipes**
   4. **Congenital dislocation of the hip**
   5. **Rhesus isoimmunisation**
   6. **Neonatal respiratory distress syndrome (RDS)**
   7. **Antepartum haemorrhage**

19.3 What is an alternative procedure to amniocentesis which yields a quicker cell culture for karyotyping? [Marks 1]
   Chorionic villus sampling/biopsy

19.4 After explaining the result to Mrs MR, what intervention should be discussed? [Marks 1]
   Termination of pregnancy

19.5 List three medical methods which may be used to perform this intervention. [Marks 3]
1. Intra-amniotic prostaglandin $F_2\alpha$
2. Extra-amniotic prostaglandin E_2
3. Vaginal prostaglandin analogue/gemeprost

STATION 20   ANSWERS   **CIRCUIT A**

20.1 What are the causes of large for dates? Name five. [Marks 5]
1. Maternal obesity
2. Adnexal pathology
3. Uterine fibroids
4. Multiple pregnancy
5. Fetal abnormality
6. Macrosomic fetus
7. Hydropic fetus
8. Polyhydramnios

20.2 Name three investigations you would perform. [Marks 3]
1. USS
2. Red cell tolerance test
3. Antibodies (to check for isoimmunisation)

20.3 What is the measurement called? [Marks 1]
Symphysiofundal height

20.4 What is its relevance? [Marks 1]
One centimetre corresponds to 1 week of gestation. (It is more useful if performed by the same examiner each time.)

CIRCUIT B

Mrs PP had a Ventouse extraction 4 days ago. She had experienced spontaneous rupture of membranes 20 hours prior to augmentation with Syntocinon. The total length of her labour was 16 hours and the placenta was noted to be irregular in one area. She is feeling feverish with cramping abdominal pain. Her observation chart is shown.

1.1   Describe three abnormal features shown on her chart.

1.2   The lochia is offensive. On examination, the uterus is 16 weeks size and tender with a patulous cervical os. What is your working diagnosis? Name two features.

1.3   List three investigations you would arrange.

1.4   In general terms, what medical treatment would you start?

1.5   Which operative procedure may be necessary?

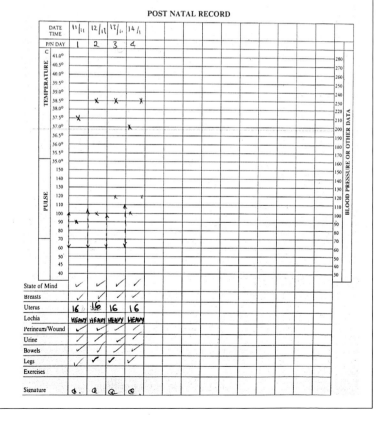

POST NATAL RECORD

Mrs MG is in the ninth week of her pregnancy. She has experienced severe nausea and vomiting over the last 3 weeks and light vaginal bleeding over the last 24 hours. A transvaginal ultrasound scan has been performed and a photograph of the findings is shown.

2.1   Describe the appearances of the uterine cavity (two features).

2.2   From the appearance of the scan, what is the likely placentation?

2.3   Two active fetal hearts are seen and the cervix is closed. What is the diagnosis?

2.4   Which two factors contribute to anaemia in this pregnancy?

2.5   Name two factors which predispose to multiple pregnancy.

2.6   Can the zygosity be predicted from the USS findings?

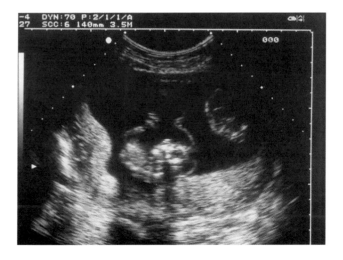

3.1 In the photograph, which structure in the neonatal skull is being examined?

3.2 Which pairs of bones form the boundaries of this structure? Name two.

3.3 If the skin over this structure is sunken, what should you suspect?

3.4 If the skin over this structure is very tense, what does this suggest?

3.5 At what age does this structure usually close?

3.6 What is the term given to a subperiosteal haematoma of the neonatal skull?

3.7 What clinical feature is pathognomonic of this?

3.8 List two complications of the above condition (Q. 3.6).

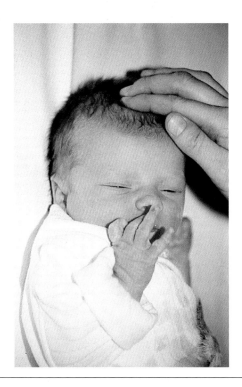

4.1 Name the two intrauterine contraceptive devices (IUCDs) illustrated.

4.2 Name three ways that these may provide contraception.

4.3 When should each of these be changed?

4.4 Name two complications of their use.

4.5 Name two absolute contraindications to the device on the right.

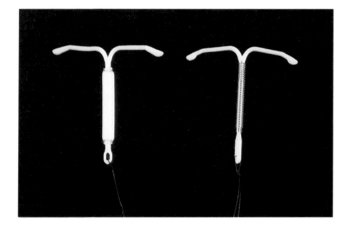

5.1   What organisms are seen on the smear?

5.2   What is the diagnosis?

5.3   Name two common symptoms of this condition.

5.4   On speculum examination, what would you expect to see?

5.5   Name three swabs you would take.

5.6   Name two treatments.

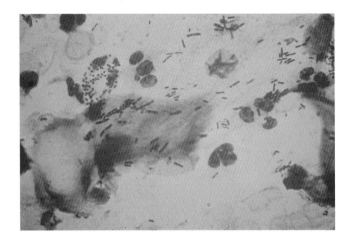

6.1 Define perinatal mortality rate (PNMR).

6.2 What is the national PNMR in the UK?

6.3 What are the major determinants of perinatal mortality? Specify three.

6.4 At what maternal age is the perinatal mortality rate at its lowest?

6.5 A report of a regular confidential enquiry is shown in the photograph. Which areas of the UK contribute to this report?

6.6 For the purposes of this report, what is the lower limit of the birthweight of babies included in the intrapartum-related deaths?

6.7 After exclusion of babies wih gross life-threatening abnormalities, which deaths in terms of timing are included in the intrapartum death group?

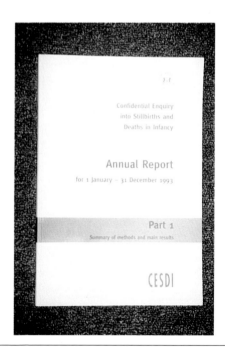

Mrs Smith is a 24-year-old woman who has reached 30 weeks gestation in her first pregnancy. Her BP was 100/65 mmHg at booking. She now has a BP of 150/95 mmHg and 3+ proteinuria. Her biochemistry is illustrated.

7.1 What specific symptoms would you ask her about? Name two.

7.2 Name three clinical signs you would look for.

7.3 What abnormal result is displayed in the biochemistry?

7.4 Where would you manage this patient?

7.5 What fetal investigations would you do? Name two.

7.6 What are the chances of this condition recurring in the next pregnancy?

Department of Clinical Chemistry St. Elsewheres NHS Trust

Surname Smith **First Name** Mary **D.O.B.** 27.03.74 **Hosp No** 123216

Consult Rymer **Ward** Antenatal **Report Date** 21.07.97

			n.r.
Sodium	135	mmol/l	(135–145)
Potassium	4.3	mmol/l	(3.5–5.0)
Urea	4.9	mmol/l	(2.5–7.5)
Creatinine	90	µmol/l	(65–101)
Alk. phosphatase	209	U/l	(38–126)
Albumin	35	g/l	(35–47)
Total protein	65	g/l	(64–80)
Alan. transaminase	20	U/l	(<55)
Total Bilirubin	5	µmol/l	(<22)
Urate	0.40	mmol/l	(0.16–0.36)

A 35-year-old primigravida presented to the labour ward at 38 weeks gestation with constant abdominal pain, some vaginal bleeding and an irritable uterus. Her BP was 160/100 mmHg. Her FBC is shown.

8.1 What is the probable diagnosis?

8.2 What other investigations are important in the immediate management of this case? Name three.

8.3 On examination, what would the uterus feel like?

8.4 What management would you institute for the mother? Name three aspects.

8.5 If the CTG showed late decelerations in response to the uterine activity, what would you do?

8.6 With these cases, if maternal death occurs, what is the most likely cause?

Guy's Hospital Department of Haematology		
	Surname	J
	Forename	J
Date 21.10.97	Sex	F
	DOB	23.7.63
	Number	124215
Haemoglobin	12.4 g/dl	
White Cell Count	$12.4 \times 10^9/l$	
Platelets	$60 \times 10^{12}/l$	
PCV	0.42	
MCV	88 fl	

This woman presented with oligoamenorrhea.

9.1 What other symptom did she present with?

9.2 What is the likely diagnosis?

9.3 Name two hormone levels that are raised in this condition.

9.4 What serum protein is reduced?

9.5 What management would you advise, assuming she did not want to conceive? Name two aspects.

9.6 In later life, what may she be at risk of? Name one condition.

9.7 Name two histological features of the ovary.

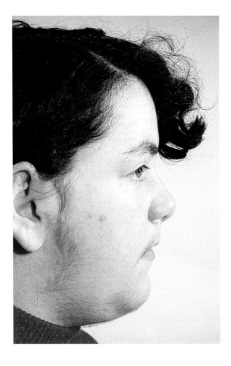

10.1 What classic symptoms may this woman have presented with? Name two.

10.2 As her GP, what would you do after receiving this report?

10.3 If the diagnosis is confirmed and is stage 1b, what is the appropriate treatment?

10.4 Name four risk factors for this disease.

10.5 What is the 5-year survival for stage 1 disease?

10.6 What age group has the highest incidence of this disease?

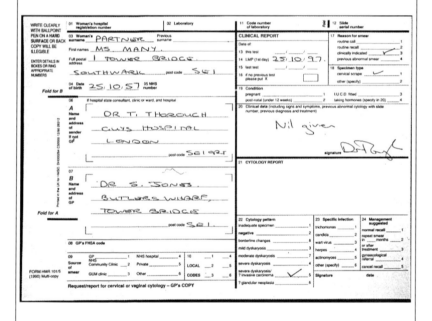

Mrs VH, age 66, had a vaginal hysterectomy 3 days ago. Her postoperative observation chart is shown.

11.1 What abnormalities can you identify? Specify two.

11.2 List four routine examinations you would perform.

11.3 List two microbiological investigations you would arrange.

11.4 Vaginal examination reveals marked tenderness of the vault. A transvaginal ultrasound report demonstrated a 7 cm × 8 cm × 10 cm collection of fluid behind the bladder containing a few bright echoes. Neither ovary was seen.

What is the likely diagnosis?

11.5 What is the usual outcome?

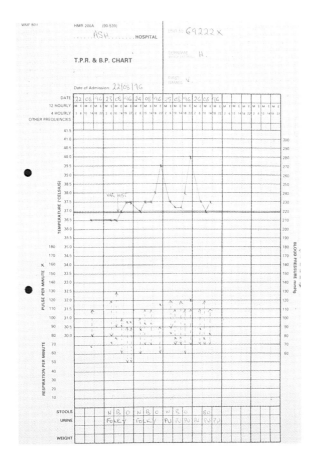

Mrs VP is a 63-year-old widow. She has been menopausal since the age of 50 and has not been sexually active since the death of her husband 8 years ago. She presents with a 6 month history of itching in the vulval area. A photograph of her vulva is shown.

12.1 Describe the appearances of the vulva. Name two features.

12.2 What is the likely diagnosis?

12.3 How would you confirm your clinical diagnosis?

12.4 What is the first line of treatment? Name two preparations.

12.5 What other local treatment may improve symptoms? Name two.

12.6 List two radical treatments which may be used to treat severe intractable vulval pruritus.

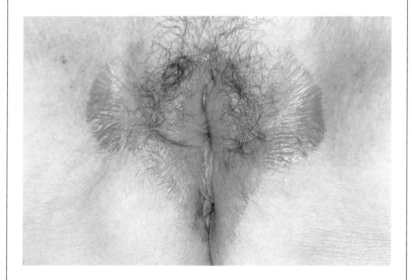

This 35-year-old woman presented with a 10 day history of pain and swelling in the right side of the vulva. The pain is throbbing and walking has become increasingly difficult. She also has an offensive vaginal discharge.

13.1 Which structure is involved?

13.2 What is the usual function of this structure?

13.3 What is the diagnosis?

13.4 How does this occur? State two mechanisms.

13.5 What are the principles of treatment? Name two.

13.6 What is this process called?

13.7 A swab from the pus drained shows Gram-negative intracellular diplococci. Where should the patient be referred?

13.8 Who else should be investigated?

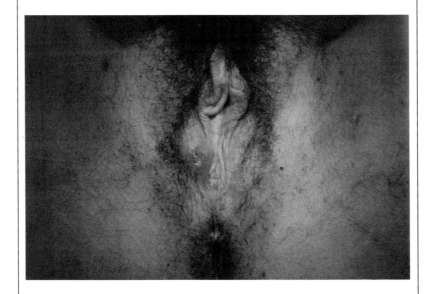

14.1 Define urinary incontinence. Specify two features.

14.2 A subtraction cystometric trace is shown. Name the abnormality which is demonstrated.

14.3 How may a woman with this result present? Specify two symptoms.

14.4 What simple measures may improve symptoms? Specify two.

14.5 Which class of drugs may be of benefit?

14.6 Give an example of this class of drug (generic name with usual dose).

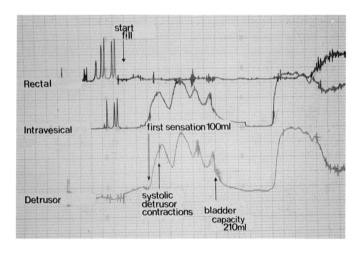

The photograph shows some commonly used preparations.

15.1 What is the generic term given to this group of preparations?

15.2 List two absolute contraindications to this treatment.

15.3 What are the long-term unseen benefits of such treatment? Name two.

15.4 What is the recommended minimum duration of therapy if long-term benefits are to be achieved?

15.5 In the non-hysterectomised woman, what are the alternatives to oral progestogen? Name two routes of administration.

15.6 What is meant by tachyphylaxis?

15.7 When using implants, how might you reduce tachyphylaxis?

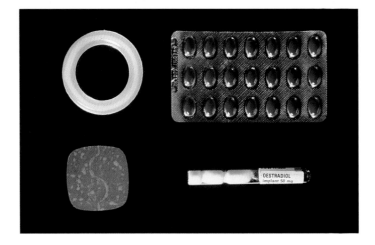

A gestational diabetic woman at term with a known large baby has been in the second stage of labour for 2 hours and you have been called to the room as she is delivering. When you walk into the room, the midwife says that she is unable to deliver all of the head. You look at the perineum and see a very blue face and make an instant diagnosis.

16.1 What is the diagnosis?

16.2 Mechanically, what has occurred?

16.3 What do you do? Name three important manoeuvres.

16.4 If these initial manoeuvres do not result in delivery, list what you would do. Name two courses of action.

16.5 If this fails, what would you do to the fetus?

16.6 If this fails, what would you do to the mother?

16.7 What would you advise for the next pregnancy if the baby is the same size or larger?

Mrs RM is in her third pregnancy. At her 38 week antenatal check by her midwife, she reports reduced fetal movements and her midwife advises her to fill in a kick chart.

17.1 What does the kick chart show?

17.2 List five causes of reduced fetal movements.

17.3 What non-invasive tests could you arrange for this woman to assess the well-being of her baby? List four tests.

- 13 -

FETAL MOVEMENT CHART

All Saints' Hospital
Tel: 01634 407311

Name ......MRS......R. M...........................

Address ....

Telephone ....

THE REASON FOR THIS CHART: This chart is to help us assess the health of your baby by finding out how active it is.
At least 10 movements should be felt each day.

INSTRUCTIONS: 1. Start at 9.00am
2. When a movement is felt, make a tick in the box under 1st, 2nd, 3rd, etc. Several movements together should be classed as one.
3. Write down the time of the 10th movement.
4. If 10 movements are not felt by 6 pm ring All Saints' Hospital and ask to speak to the Liaison Midwife. She will make arrangements to monitor your baby.

START 9.00 AM

MOVEMENT OR KICKS

Date:	1st	2nd	3rd	4th	5th	6th	7th	8th	9th	10th+
Fri										
Sat										
Sun										
Mon										
11/9 Tue	✓	✓	✓	✓	✓	✓	✓		✓	1.30 PM
12/9 Wed	✓	✓	✓	✓	✓	✓	✓		✓	12.30 PM
13/9 Thu	✓	✓	✓	✓	✓	✓	✓		✓	1.00 PM
14/9 Fri	✓	✓	✓	✓	✓	✓			✓	3.30 PM
15/9 Sat	✓	✓	✓	✓	✓	✓9.00 PM				
Sun										
Mon										
Tue										
Wed										
Thu										

OUCHI

GOAL!

A partogram is shown of a woman in her first labour.

18.1 When should charting of observations on a partogram be commenced?

18.2 What two criteria must be satisfied to make this diagnosis?

18.3 What abnormality is illustrated in the first stage of labour?

18.4 What intervention has been applied at A?

18.5 What has happened as a result of this intervention? State two consequences.

18.6 What is the minimum acceptable rate of cervical dilatation in the active phase of labour in a primiparous woman?

18.7 What other abnormality is illustrated?

18.8 How was this managed?

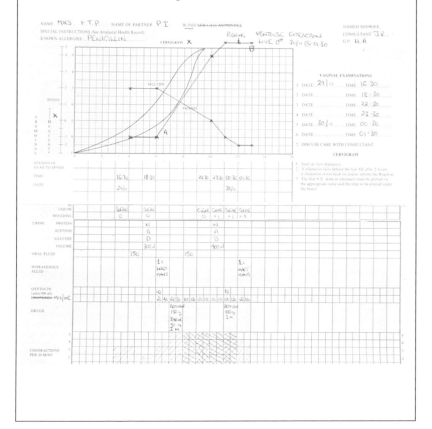

Look at investigation A.

19.1 What is this investigation called?

19.2 The subject is in her first pregnancy. Look at the abdominal X-ray (B). Why do you think investigation A has been performed?

19.3 What other investigations would you request to aid in the decision regarding the mode of delivery? Name the investigation and two parameters.

19.4 Prior to attempting a vaginal delivery at term in a primigravida with a breech presentation, what should the maximum estimated fetal weight be?

19.5 Prior to attempting a vaginal delivery at term in a primigravida with a breech presentation, what should the minimum anteroposterior pelvic inlet diameter be?

19.6 In such a case, what should be the minimum rate of cervical dilatation in the active phase of labour?

19.7 Name two other methods of assessing pelvic capacity.

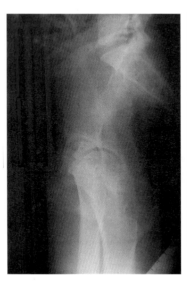 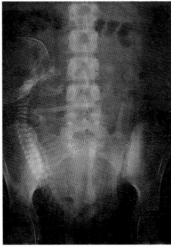

Mrs GD is 32 years old and in her fourth pregnancy. In her first pregnancy 14 years ago, she had an unexplained intrauterine death at 36 weeks. She has subsequently had two sons, aged 12 and 6, both by spontaneous vaginal delivery, weighing 4.2 and 4.6 kg at birth, respectively. At the 24 and 26 week antenatal visit, she had 2+ of glucose on urine analysis. Mrs GD's mother had maturity onset non-insulin-dependent diabetes. A 28 week, 75 g oral glucose tolerance test result is shown.

20.1 What is the diagnosis?

20.2 List four indications for a glucose tolerance test in Mrs GD's history.

20.3 Which blood test would reflect long-term glycaemia in this woman?

20.4 Name three other personnel whom you would involve in Mrs GD's management.

20.5 How would you control Mrs GD's glycaemia in labour?

Guy's Hospital
Department of Biochemistry

Date 11.10.97

Surname _____D_____

Forename _____G_____

Sex _____F_____

DOB _____29.11.64_____

Number _____641129_____

Time	Blood Glucose
Fasting	4.9 mmol/l
60 minutes	11.3 mmol/l
120 minutes	15.1 mmol/l

1.1 Describe three abnormal features shown on her chart.
[Marks 3]
1. **Pyrexia 38.5°C**
2. **Tachycardia 100–120/min**
3. **Heavy vaginal loss/lochia**

1.2 The lochia is offensive. On examination, uterus is 16/40 size and tender with a patulous cervical os. What is your working diagnosis? Name two features. [Marks 2]
1. **Retained products of conception**
2. **Endometritis**

1.3 List three investigations you would arrange. [Marks 3]
1. **Midstream urine for culture and sensitivity**
2. **Blood culture**
3. **White cell count**
4. **Endocervical swab/high vaginal swab**

1.4 In general terms, what medical treatment would you start?
[Marks 1]
Broad spectrum antibiotics

1.5 Which operative procedure may be necessary? [Marks 1]
Evacuation of retained products of conception

2.1 Describe the appearances of the uterine cavity (two features). [Marks 2]
There are two intrauterine gestation sacs, each containing a fetal pole.

2.2 From the appearance on the scan, what is the likely placentation? [Marks 2]
Dichorionic, diamniotic

2.3 Two active fetal hearts are seen and the cervix is closed. What is the diagnosis? [Marks 1]
Threatened miscarriage/threatened abortion

2.4 Which two factors contribute to anaemia in this pregnancy? [Marks 2]
1. **Increased plasma volume**
2. **Decreased red cell concentration**
3. **Increased haematinic demand**

2.5 Name two factors which predispose to multiple pregnancy. [Marks 2]
1. **Increased maternal age**
2. **Positive family history**
3. **Ovulation induction/assisted conception**

2.6 Can the zygosity be predicted from the USS findings? [Marks 1]
No

3.1 In the photograph, which structure in the neonatal skull is being examined? [Marks 1]
The anterior fontanelle/bregma

3.2 Which pairs of bones form the boundaries of this structure? Name two. [Marks 2]
Frontal and parietal bones

3.3 If the skin over this structure is sunken, what should you suspect? [Marks 1]
Neonatal dehydration

3.4 If the skin over this structure is very tense, what does this suggest? [Marks 1]
Increased intracranial tension/ hydrocephalus/meningitis

3.5 At what age does this structure usually close? [Marks 1]
6 months

3.6 What is the term given to a subperiosteal haematoma of the neonatal skull? [Marks 1]
Cephalhaematoma

3.7 What clinical feature is pathognomonic of this? [Marks 1]
Haematoma that does not cross the suture lines

3.8 List two complications of the above condition (Q. 3.6). [Marks 2]
1. **Neonatal shock/anaemia**
2. **Neonatal jaundice**

4.1 Name the two IUCDs illustrated. [Marks 2]
1. **Mirena – progestagen containing IUCD**
2. **Nova T**

4.2 Name two ways that these may provide contraception. [Marks 2]
1. **Preventing implantation**
2. **Promoting hostile cervical mucus**
3. **Impeding sperm transport**

4.3 When should each of these be changed? [Marks 2]
1. **3 years**
2. **5 years**

4.4 Name two complications of their use. [Marks 2]
1. **Pelvic infection**
2. **Expulsion**
3. **Perforation**

4.5 Name two absolute contraindications to the device on the right. [Marks 2]
1. **Copper allergy (Wilson's disease)**
2. **PID**
3. **Past history of tubal ectopic pregnancy in nulliparous women**
4. **Distorted uterine activity**

5.1 What organisms are seen on the smear? [Marks 1]
Gram-negative diplococci

5.2 What is the diagnosis? [Marks 1]
Gonorrhoea

5.3 Name two common symptoms of this condition. [Marks 2]
1. **Vaginal discharge**
2. **Dysuria**

5.4 On speculum examination, what would you expect to see? [Marks 1]
Mucopurulent cervical discharge

5.5 Name three swabs you would take. [Marks 3]
1. **Endocervix**
2. **Urethra**
3. **Rectum**
4. **Pharynx**

5.6 Name two treatments. [Marks 2]
1. **Aqueous procaine penicillin 2.4–4.8 mu i.m. with or without probenecid 1 g orally**
2. **Spectinomycin 2–4 g i.m.**
3. **Ampicillin 3 g orally with probenecid 1 g**
4. **Cefadroxil 1 g by mouth**
5. **Ciprofloxacin 500 g**
6. **Doxcycline 300 mg by mouth**
7. **Minocycline 300 mg by mouth**

STATION 6	ANSWERS	CIRCUIT B

6.1 Define perinatal mortality rate (PNMR). [Marks 1]
The number stillbirths and first week neonatal deaths per 1000 total births

6.2 What is the national PNMR in the UK? [Marks 1]
8–9 per 1000 total births

6.3 What are the major determinants of perinatal mortality? Specify three. [Marks 3]
1. **Congenital abnormality**
2. **Low birth weight**
3. **Asphyxia**

6.4 At what maternal age is the perinatal mortality rate at its lowest? [Marks 1]
20–24 years

6.5 A report of a regular confidential enquiry is shown in the photograph. Which areas of the UK contribute to this report? [Marks 3]
England, Wales and Northern Ireland

6.6 For the purposes of this report, what is the lower limit of the birthweight of babies included in the intrapartum-related deaths? [Marks 1]
2500 g

6.7 After exclusion of babies with gross life-threatening abnormalities, which deaths in terms of timing are included in the intrapartum death group? [Marks 2]
Deaths occurring in labour or within up to 6 completed days of life

STATION 7	ANSWERS	CIRCUIT B

7.1 What specific symptoms would you ask her about? Name two. [Marks 2]
1. **Nausea, vomiting**
2. **Epigastric pain**
3. **Visual symptoms**
4. **Headache**

7.2 Name three clinical signs you would look for. [Marks 3]
1. **Hyperreflexia**
2. **Clonus**
3. **Hepatic tenderness**
4. **Optic fundi changes**
5. **Hand, and facial oedema**

7.3 What abnormal result is displayed in the biochemistry? [Marks 1]
High serum urate

7.4 Where would you manage this patient? [Marks 1]
In hospital

7.5 What fetal investigations would you do? Name two. [Marks 2]
1. **Cardiotocograph (CTG)**
2. **USS**
3. **Doppler studies**
4. **Biophysical profile**

7.6 What are the chances of this condition recurring in the next pregnancy? [Marks 1]
Very low, < 5%

STATION 8	ANSWERS	CIRCUIT B

8.1 What is the probable diagnosis? [Marks 1]
Placental abruption

8.2 What other investigations are important in the immediate management of this case? [Marks 3]
1. **Clotting studies**
2. **U+E urate**
3. **Urine for protein**
4. **CTG**

8.3 On examination, what would the uterus feel like? [Marks 1]
Wood hard/tense

8.4 What management would you institute for the mother? Name three aspects. [Marks 3]
1. **IV line/IV fluids**
2. **Blood for cross match**
3. **Urinary catheter**
4. **Resuscitation if needed**

8.5 If the CTG showed late decelerations in response to the uterine activity, what would you do? [Marks 1]
Institute delivery

8.6 With these cases, if maternal death occurs, what is the most likely cause? [Marks 1]
DIC

STATION 9 ANSWERS   **CIRCUIT B**

9.1 What other symptom did she present with? [Marks 1]
Hirsutism

9.2 What is the likely diagnosis? [Marks 1]
PCOS

9.3 Name two hormone levels that are raised in this condition. [Marks 2]
1. **Luteinising hormone (LH)**
2. **Testosterone**
3. **Oestrogen**
4. **Androstenedione**
5. **Dihydroepiandosterone (DHEA)**

9.4 What serum protein is reduced? [Marks 1]
Sex hormone binding globulin (SHBG)

9.5 What management would you advise, assuming she did not want to conceive? Name two aspects. [Marks 2]
1. **Ethinyl oestradiol and cyproterone acetate**
2. **Dianette/low androgenic OC pill**
3. **Advise weight reduction**

9.6 In later life, what may she be at risk of? Name one condition. [Marks 1]
1. **Endometrial pathology**
2. **Cardiovascular disease**

9.7 Name two histological features of the ovary. [Marks 2]
1. **Thick smooth pearly white capsule**
2. **Multiple small peripherally placed follicles**
3. **Thecal cell hyperplasia**

STATION 10	ANSWERS	CIRCUIT B

10.1 What classic symptoms may this woman have presented with? Name two. [Marks 2]
1. **Postcoital bleeding**
2. **Intermenstrual bleeding**

10.2 As her GP, what would you do after receiving this report? [Marks 1]
1. **Refer immediately for colposcopy**
2. **Refer to gynaecologist for biopsy**

10.3 If the diagnosis is confirmed and is stage 1b, what is the appropriate treatment? [Marks 1]
Wertheim's hysterectomy or radiotherapy

10.4 Name four risk factors for this disease. [Marks 4]
1. **Large number of sexual partners**
2. **HPV 16 and 18**
3. **Smoking**
4. **Previous cervical intraepithelial neoplasia (CIN)**
5. **History of sexually transmitted disease (STD)**
6. **Early age of first coitus**

10.5 What is the 5-year survival for stage 1 disease? [Marks 1]
80%

10.6 What age group has the highest incidence of this disease? [Marks 1]
50–60 years

11.1 What abnormalities can you identify? Specify two. [Marks 2]
1. **Swinging pyrexia**
2. **Tachycardia with pyrexia**

11.2 List four routine examinations you would perform. [Marks 4]
1. **Examine the respiratory system/exclude pneumonia or atelectasis**
2. **Examine the legs/exclude deep venous thrombosis**
3. **Examine the wound/exclude wound infection, wound abscess**
4. **Examine the vaginal vault/exclude vault haematoma**
5. **Ballot kidneys/exclude pyelonephritis**

11.3 List two microbiological investigations you would arrange. [Marks 2]
1. **Midstream urine for culture and sensitivity**
2. **Wound swab for microscopy, culture and sensitivity**
3. **Blood for culture and sensitivity**
4. **High vaginal swab for microscopy culture and sensitivity**

11.4 Vaginal examination reveals marked tenderness of the vault. A transvaginal ultrasound is carried out (see report). What is the likely diagnosis? [Marks 1]
Infected vault haematoma

11.5 What is the usual outcome? [Marks 1]
Spontaneous drainage/resolution

| **STATION 12** ANSWERS | **CIRCUIT B** |

12.1 Describe the appearances of the vulva. Name two features. [Marks 2]
Papery thin atrophic areas interspersed with reddened thick areas

12.2 What is the likely diagnosis? [Marks 2]
Lichen sclerosis et atrophicus

12.3 How would you confirm your clinical diagnosis? [Marks 1]
Skin biopsy and histological analysis/examination

12.4 What is the first line of treatment? Name two preparations. [Marks 2]
1. **Topical glucocorticoids/hydrocortisone**
2. **Dermovate/betnovate/betamethasone**

12.5 What other local treatment may improve symptoms? Name two. [Marks 2]
Topical oestrogen cream/local anaesthetic/topical 2% testosterone

12.6 List two radical treatments which may be used to treat severe intractable vulval pruritus. [Marks 2]
1. **Radiotherapy**
2. **Skinning vulvectomy/simple vulvectomy**

| **STATION 13** | ANSWERS | **CIRCUIT B** |

13.1 Which structure is involved? [Marks 1]
Bartholin's gland

13.2 What is the usual function of this structure? [Marks 1]
Secretion of mucoid fluid for lubrication

13.3 What is the diagnosis? [Marks 1]
Bartholin's abscess

13.4 How does this occur? State two mechanisms. [Marks 2]
1. **Duct of Bartholin's gland becomes blocked**
2. **Mucoid secretion collects and becomes infected**

13.5 What are the principles of treatment? Name two. [Marks 2]
1. **Deroofing the Bartholin's abscess to drain off pus**
2. **Maintaining duct patency to encourage ongoing drainage**

13.6 What is this process called? [Marks 1]
Marsupialisation

13.7 A swab from the pus drained shows Gram-negative intracellular diplococci. Where should the patient be reffered? [Marks 1]
Genitourinary medicine clinic/STD clinic

13.8 Who else should be investigated? [Marks 1]
The woman's partner(s)

14.1 Define urinary incontinence. [Marks 1]
This is a condition in which there is involuntary loss of urine, leading to a social or personal problem with hygiene

14.2 A subtraction cystometric trace is shown. Name the abnormality which is demonstrated. [Marks 1]
Detrusor instability

14.3 How may a woman with this result present? Specify two symptoms. [Marks 2]
1. **Stress incontinence/urge incontinence**
2. **Frequency/urgency/dysuria**
3. **Nocturia/enuresis**

14.4 What simple measures may improve symptoms? Specify two. [Marks 2]
1. **Bladder drill/bladder training**
2. **Reduction in fluid intake, especially in the evening**
3. **Avoidance of caffeine**

14.5 Which class of drugs may be of benefit? [Marks 1]
Anticholinergic drugs

14.6 Give an example of this class of drug (generic name with usual dose). [Marks 2]
1. **Propantheline hydrochloride 15 mg B.D.**
2. **Oxybutynin 2.5 mg B.D.**
3. **Imipramine 25 mg daily**

15.1 What is the generic term given to this group of preparations? [Marks 1]
Hormone replacement therapy

15.2 List two absolute contraindications to this treatment. [Marks 2]
1. **Oestrogen-dependent tumour/breast carcinoma/endometrial carcinoma**
2. **Active liver disease/chronic active hepatitis/acute hepatitis**
3. **Undiagnosed abnormal vaginal bleeding**

15.3 What are the long-term unseen benefits of such treatment? Name two. [Marks 2]

1. **Prevention of osteoporosis/bone loss/preservation of bone**
2. **Prevention of coronary heart disease/myocardial infarction**
3. **Prevention of Alzheimer's**
4. **Prevention of cerebrovascular accidents**
5. **Prevention of colorectal cancer**

15.4 What is the recommended minimum duration of therapy if long-term benefits are to be achieved? [Marks 1]
At least 5 years

15.5 In the non-hysterectomised woman, what are the alternatives to oral progestogen? Name two routes of administration. [Marks 2]

1. **Transdermal progestogen**
2. **Intrauterine progestogen-containing device**

15.6 What is meant by tachyphylaxis? [Marks 1]
Return of symptoms despite high levels of drug/oestrogen

15.7 When using implants, how might you reduce tachyphylasis? [Marks 1]

1. **Measure serum oestradiol prior to administration**
2. **Strict adherence to time of giving implants (i.e. not less than 6 months apart).**

<table>
<tr><td>STATION 16</td><td>ANSWERS</td><td>CIRCUIT B</td></tr>
</table>

16.1 What is the diagnosis? [Marks 1]
Shoulder dystocia

16.2 Mechanically, what has occurred? [Marks 1]
The shoulders have impacted on the symphysis pubis

16.3 What do you do? Name three important manoeuvres. [Marks 3]

1. **Lithotomy position/left lateral position**
2. **Large episiotomy**
3. **Ask for suprapubic pressure**

16.4 If these initial manoeuvres do not result in delivery, list what you would do. Name two courses of action. [Marks 2]

1. **Convert shoulders into diagonal position**
2. **Deliver posterior shoulder**

OSCEs IN OBSTETRICS AND GYNAECOLOGY

16.5 If this fails, what would you do to the fetus? [Marks 1]
Break the clavicles

16.6 If this fails, what would you do to the mother? [Marks 1]
Symphysiotomy

16.7 What would you advise for the next pregnancy if the baby is the same size or larger? [Marks 1]
Elective LSCS

STATION 17 ANSWERS   **CIRCUIT B**

17.1 What does the kick chart show? [Marks 1]
Reduced fetal movements: six movements in 12 hours

17.2 List five causes of reduced fetal movements. [Marks 5]
1. **Normal sleep phase**
2. **Physiological (towards the end of pregnancy)**
3. **Reduced maternal perception (idiopathic or due to distraction)**
4. **Sedative drugs given to mother (e.g. barbiturates)**
5. **Polyhydramnios/oligohydramnios**
6. **Intrauterine asphyxia**

17.3 What non-invasive tests could you arrange for this woman to assess the well-being of her baby? List four tests. [Marks 4]
1. **Cardiotocography (non-stress)**
2. **Ultrasound for fetal growth and liquor**
3. **Formal biophysical profile**
4. **Umbilical artery Doppler studies/velocimetry**

STATION 18 ANSWERS   **CIRCUIT B**

18.1 When should charting of observations on a partogram be commenced? [Marks 1]
1. **When labour is established/has reached the active phase**
2. **When diagnosis of labour has been made**

18.2 What two criteria must be satisfied to make this diagnosis? [Marks 2]
Regular uterine contractions accompanied by progressive cervical change

18.3 What abnormality is illustrated in the first stage of labour? [Marks 1]
Primary uterine inertia/prolonged first stage/delayed progress in first stage/primary arrest

18.4 What intervention has been applied at A? [Marks 1]
Oxytocin infusion

18.5 What has happened as a result of this intervention? State two consequences. [Marks 2]
1. **Increase in intensity/frequency/duration of contractions**
2. **Acceleration of cervical dilatation**

18.6 What is the minimum acceptable rate of cervical dilatation in the active phase of labour in a primiparous woman? [Marks 1]
More than or equal to 1 cm/hour

18.7 What other abnormality is illustrated? [Marks 1]
Secondary arrest/prolonged second stage

18.8 How was this managed? [Marks 1]
Ventouse extraction/operative vaginal delivery

STATION 19	ANSWERS		CIRCUIT B

19.1 What is this investigation called? [Marks 1]
An erect lateral pelvimetry

19.2 The subject is in her first pregnancy. Why do you think the investigation has been performed? [Marks 1]
Because of breech presentation

19.3 What other investigations would you request to aid in the decision regarding the mode of delivery? Name the investigation and two parameters. [Marks 3]
1. **Ultrasound scan to estimate the fetal weight**
2. **Ultrasound scan to assess the fetal attitude**

19.4 Prior to attempting a vaginal delivery at term in a primipara with a breech presentation, what should the maximum estimated fetal weight be? [Marks 1]
3.5 kg

OSCEs IN OBSTETRICS AND GYNAECOLOGY

19.5 Prior to attempting a vaginal delivery at term in a primipara with a breech presentation, what should the minimum anteroposterior pelvic inlet diameter be? [Marks 1]
11.5 cm

19.6 In such a case, what should be the minimum rate of cervical dilatation in the active phase of labour? [Marks 1]
Greater than or equal to 1 cm/hour; at least 1 cm/hour

19.7 Name two other methods of assessing pelvic capacity. [Marks 2]
1. **Clinical/digital pelvimetry**
2. **CT pelvimetry/magnetic resonance imaging (MRI)**

STATION 20	ANSWERS	CIRCUIT B

20.1 What is the diagnosis? [Marks 1]
Diabetes mellitus in pregnancy

20.2 List four indications for a glucose tolerance test in Mrs GD's history. [Marks 4]
1. **Family history of diabetes mellitus**
2. **Unexplained IUD**
3. **Previous fetal macrosomia**
4. **Persistent glycosuria**

20.3 Which blood test would reflect long-term glycaemia in this woman? [Marks 1]
Glycosolated haemoglobin/haemoglobin A1C/fructosamine

20.4 Name three other personnel whom you would involve in Mrs GD's management. [Marks 3]
1. **Consultant endocrinologist/diabetologist**
2. **Diabetic specialist nurse/midwife**
3. **Dietician**

20.5 How would you control Mrs GD's glycaemia in labour? [Marks 1]
Continuous glucose infusion together with sliding scale insulin infusion

CIRCUIT C

1.1 Name four advantages of the method of contraception shown below.

1.2 Name four disadvantages.

1.3 If this method failed during intercourse, what would you advise for emergency contraception? Name constituents.

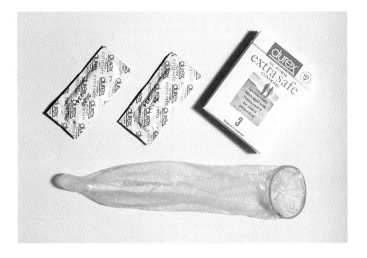

Mrs AM is 39 weeks pregnant in her third pregnancy. Her antenatal hepatitis B screening result is shown.

2.1 Specify four mechanisms by which hepatitis B infection may be transmitted.

2.2 What grade of infectivity does the blood result imply?

2.3 What three measures would you recommend for this woman's newborn baby?

2.4 How soon should the newborn baby be immunized?

2.5 Of those babies infected perinatally, what percentage will become chronic carriers?

Guy's Hospital **Department of Virology**	Surname _____ M _____
	Forename _____ A _____
Date 19.7.97	Sex _____ F _____
	DOB _____ 2.2.58 _____
	Number _____ S80202 _____
Hepatitis B surface antigen detected e antigen detected e antibody negative	

The table shows deaths from hypertensive disorders of pregnancy in the UK between 1985 and 1993.

3.1 Comment on the two trends shown.

3.2 In 1991–1993, substandard care was identified in 80% of cases. How does this compare with previous triennia?

3.3 Two factors have consistently been identified as contributing to the substandard care. What are these?

3.4 In 1991–1993, 11 deaths followed eclampsia. In none of these cases was magnesium sulphate used. How may this change and why?

3.5 Give three recommendations made at the end of the 1991–1993 report with regard to hypertensive disease in pregnancy.

The number of women who died from hypertensive disorders of pregnancy in the 3 triennia from 1985 to 1993		
Triennium	Number of deaths	Death rate (per million pregnancies)
1985–1987	27	12.1
1988–1990	27	11.0
1991–1993	20	8.6
Adapted from Maternal Mortality Report 1991–1993, Department of Health		

Mrs EF has been attending your GP surgery for her antenatal care and her antenatal records are shown.

4.1 With regards to BP in pregnancy, what normally happens in the first trimester?

4.2 What happens in the second trimester normally?

4.3 What happens in the third trimester normally?

4.4 What features are you concerned about with Mrs EF? Name two.

4.5 What do you arrange now? Name three measures.

4.6 In the latest maternal mortality report (1991–1993), where did hypertensive diseases rate among the commonest causes of direct deaths?

4.7 In deaths from hypertensive disease, what was the commonest cause?

Mrs EF LMP 6/12/96		Antenatal Record EDD 12/9/97								DOB 10/1/65
Date	Gestation	Problems	SFH	Position	Descent of head	Fetal heart	BP	Urine Prot. ClU.	Comment	Seen by & date
27/2/97	11	—	—	—	—	—	$\frac{110}{70}$	– –	Delighted	2/4
2/4/97	16	Nil	—	—	—	—	$\frac{100}{60}$	– –	Tired	25/4
25/4/97	20	Nil	20 cm	—	—	Heard	$\frac{110}{60}$	– –	Feels fine	22/5
22/5/97	24	Nil	24 cm	—	—	Heard	$\frac{120}{70}$	– –	All well	21/6
21/6/97	28	Nil	27 cm	Ceph.	5/5	Heard	$\frac{120}{70}$	– ·–	Fine	19/7
19/7/97	32	Tired	31 cm	Ceph.	4/5	Heard	$\frac{150}{95}$	1+ –		

You are called to the labour ward 15 minutes after a para 3 gravida 4 has had a normal delivery. She is bleeding excessively.

5.1   What is the first thing you do when you enter the room (apart from introducing yourself).

5.2   What two relevant questions do you ask the midwife?

5.3   What do you then do? Name five courses of action.

5.4   What is the most likely cause?

5.5   You are unable to stop the bleeding. What measure do you take while awaiting senior help?

Part of Ms HP's antenatal care chart is shown.

6.1 List five features that place her in a high-risk category for pregnancy which would have been identified at the booking visit.

6.2 Comment on her 24 and 26 weeks visits to her midwife.

6.3 What investigation would you have arranged?

6.4 She is seen in the hospital antenatal clinic around 32/40. Comment on the abdominal findings.

6.5 What investigation would you arrange at this visit?

6.6 At 38/40, Ms HP is delivered of a 2.1 kg baby boy by LSCS. Comment on this.

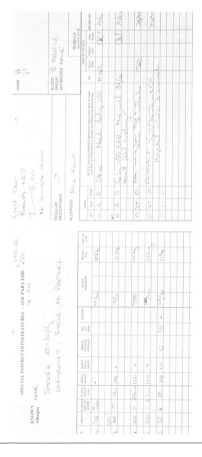

Mrs PB had a Neville–Barnes forceps delivery for a prolonged second stage in her first pregnancy 6 days ago. She has been suffering with perineal pain since the delivery, which has not improved, and it continues to be painful to sit or open her bowels. A photograph of her perineum is shown.

7.1 What has happened?

7.2 List four factors which may predispose to this complication.

7.3 In the absence of infection, how is this complication best managed? Specify two points.

7.4 List three simple measures which may improve symptoms.

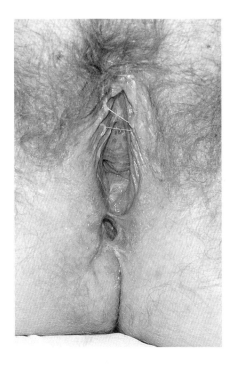

A 19-year-old girl presents with primary amenorrhoea. She has a webbed neck and a wide carrying angle. She is 141 cm. A X-ray of her hands is shown.

8.1   What abnormality is shown?

8.2   What is the most likely diagnosis?

8.3   If you analysed her chromosomes, what would they show?

8.4   What hormone test would you request?

8.5   What would her uterus look like?

8.6   What would her gonads look like?

8.7   What hormonal replacement would you give her?

8.8   Name two conditions under which this woman could become pregnant.

8.9   Name one way this condition could have been detected during her mother's pregnancy.

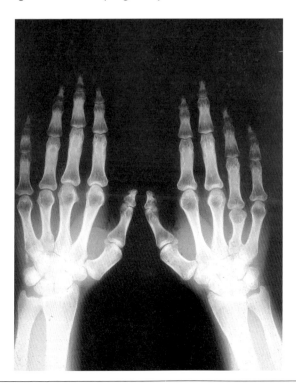

This 76-year old woman presented with soreness of the vulva.

9.1 What do you see?

9.2 What is the most likely diagnosis?

9.3 What is the most common histological diagnosis?

9.4 Which nodes would this spread to?

9.5 What is the treatment of choice? Name two components.

9.6 What is the 5-year survival rate for node negative stage 1 cases?

9.7 Name three predisposing factors for this condition.

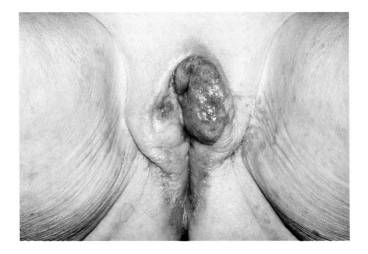

This photograph was taken laparoscopically.

10.1 What abnormality does it show?

10.2 Name three symptoms this patient may have presented with?

10.3 If she was to have this abnormality removed by a conservative procedure, what intraoperative complications may arise? Name two.

10.4 What must a patient be warned about prior to this operation?

10.5 If this woman had become pregnant prior to her operation, name two complications that she may have had during the pregnancy.

10.6 In what percentage of cases may this condition be malignant?

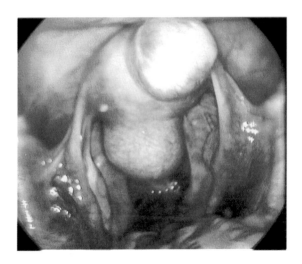

Mrs CD is a 35-year-old housewife with two children. She was sterilised 2 years ago and since the operation her periods have been very heavy. Her GP performed a cervical smear and the result is shown.

11.1 What does the result suggest?

11.2 What investigation is indicated? Name two features.

11.3 Name two solutions used to identify abnormal areas on the cervix.

11.4 The squamo-columnar junction is wholly visible and biopsy of a clearly defined abdominal area confirms CIN II. List three methods suitable for removing the abnormal area.

11.5 If the extent of the abnormal area is not visible, which diagnostic procedure is indicated?

11.6 Given Mrs CD's menstrual history, what other surgical options should be considered? Name one.

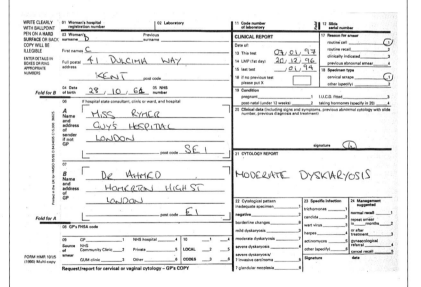

An X-ray is shown.

12.1 What is this investigation called?

12.2 Describe the findings. Specify two features.

12.3 What is the commonest microorganism leading to this picture?

12.4 In the presence of normal ovulation and a normal semen analysis in her partner, what are the two options for facilitating conception in this patient?

12.5 What is the usually quoted take-home baby rate following in vitro fertilisation in experienced hands?

12.6 List three important complications of IVF.

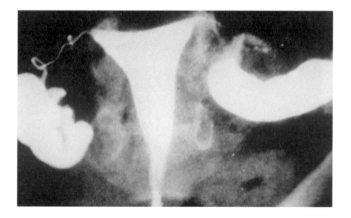

A 22-year-old woman who has recently married complained of deep dyspareunia on every occasion of coitus. She also reports a copious inoffensive discharge and occasional postcoital bleeding. She uses the combined oral contraceptive pill and has regular withdrawal bleeds.

13.1 List three investigations you would arrange during your speculum examination.

13.2 Speculum examination reveals a florid ectropion. Which of her symptoms might cause this? Name two.

13.3 If the investigations performed in Question 13.1 were normal, how would you treat the ectropion?

13.4 Name the structure shown below.

13.5 What is this used for?

13.6 Use of this structure results in the alleviation of symptoms. Which operation would you recommend?

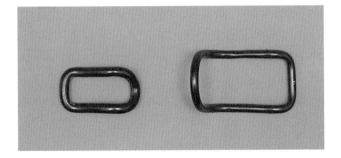

14.1 Look at the result shown. Name the investigation.

14.2 Define a normal urinary flow rate for a woman.

14.3 What is the abnormality shown?

14.4 What simple measures may improve the patient's symptoms? Name two.

14.5 List three surgical approaches to treat this condition, and provide an example of each.

14.6 Which operation has the highest documented success rate?

14.7 What is the usually quoted success rate in experienced hands?

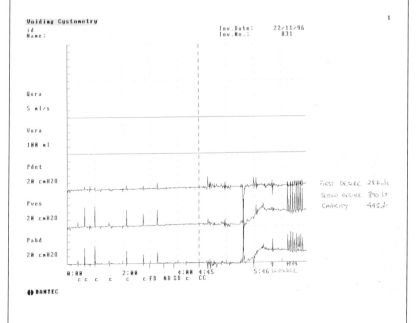

A 34-year-old lady presents to her GP at 27 weeks in her first pregnancy complaining of lower abdominal pain.

15.1 Give three possible uterine causes of the pain.

15.2 Give three possible non-uterine causes of the pain.

15.3 What clinical signs would you look for on examination to help you make a diagnosis? Name four.

This station concerns drugs in pregnancy.

16.1 Define the term teratogen.

16.2 What is the approximate molecular weight of substances which readily cross the placenta?

16.3 List the three phases of development of a conceptus and specify the precise timing in completed weeks post-conception.

16.4 At which of these phases does exposure to a teratogen have the greatest potential to cause gross malformation?

16.5 What criteria must be satisfied before prescribing a pregnant woman a known teratogen?

17.1 What is the incidence of spontaneous twins in the UK?

17.2 This incidence is rising. Why?

17.3 What percentage of spontaneous twins are monozygotic?

17.4 Graphs 1 and 2 show serial ultrasound measurements of abdominal and head circumference in a monochorionic–diamniotic twin pregnancy. Describe three findings.

17.5 Graph 3 shows serial amniotic fluid index measurements from the two sacs. Describe two findings.

17.6 What term is used to describe this sequence of events?

17.7 Umbilical arterial Doppler of twin 2 shows reversed end diastolic flow. What would you arrange?

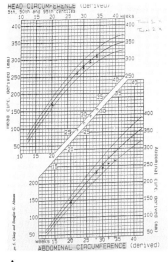

A

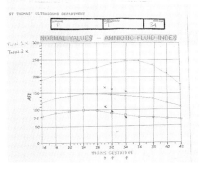

B

Miss PL is a 15-year-old schoolgirl who is 29 weeks pregnant. She has previously had an evacuation termination of pregnancy at 15 weeks gestation for social reasons. She has smoked since the age of 11 and lives with her unemployed divorced mother on income support. She presents to the labour ward with a 3 hour history of painful contractions every 10 minutes.

18.1 Define preterm delivery.

18.2 What is the incidence of preterm delivery?

18.3 List four risk factors for preterm delivery in Miss PL's history.

18.4 What examinations would you carry out to establish a diagnosis of preterm labour? Specify two.

18.5 In the presence of preterm labour, what would you administer to Miss PL to encourage fetal lung maturation? Specify preparation, dose, route of administration and frequency.

A 26-year-old woman presents to the antenatal clinic at 18 weeks gestation and the subject of HIV antenatal testing is discussed with her. She agrees to have the test as her previous partner was bisexual. The results come back positive and termination is discussed. She declines termination.

19.1 What would you advise her about the rate of vertical transmission?

19.2 During the pregnancy, her CD4 count is <200 mm^3 on three occasions. What would you give her for prophylaxis against *Pneumocystis carinii* pneumonia (PCP)?

19.3 She develops oral candidiasis. What would you give her?

19.4 This appears to be ineffective. What would you offer her?

19.5 Would you give her folic acid? Justify your answer.

19.6 What iron preparation would you give her?

19.7 Does caesarean section offer any advantage with regard to vertical transmission?

19.8 How long does it take for the baby to lose maternal antibody?

19.9 What immunisations should the baby not be given? Name two.

Miss EP was referred to A&E with a 6.5 week history of amenorrhoea and left iliac fossa pain. A urinary BHCG was positive and a transvaginal ultrasound scan was performed, shown below.

20.1 Describe the appearance of the uterine cavity.

20.2 Describe the finding to the left of the uterus.

20.3 Where is the answer to Question 20.2 likely to be located?

20.4 Miss EP is haemodynamically stable with no signs of peritonism. State four different methods of treating her condition.

20.5 If a laparoscopic conservative procedure is performed, when would you expect Miss EP to be well enough to go home?

20.6 How should she be followed up?

20.7 What is currently the most common aetiological factor associated with ectopic pregnancy?

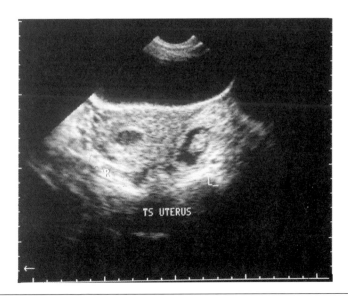

1.1 Name four advantages of the method of contraception shown below. [Marks 4]
1. **Protection against STD**
2. **Protection from carcinoma of the cervix**
3. **No systemic side effects**
4. **Easily available**
5. **Instantly effective**

1.2 Name four disadvantages. [Marks 4]
1. **Requires continuous motivation**
2. **Action required at time of coitus**
3. **User failure can be high**
4. **Decreased sensation in the male**
5. **Latex allergies**

1.3 If this method failed during intercourse, what would you advise for emergency contraception? Name constituents. [Marks 2]
Ethinyl oestradiol 50 µg and levonorgestrol 250 µg – two doses, separated by 12 hours PC4 (within 72 hours)

2.1 Specify four mechanisms by which hepatitis B infection may be transmitted. [Marks 4]
1. **Sexually/anal intercourse/vaginal intercourse**
2. **Parenterally/blood transfusion/needle stick**
3. **Perinatal transmission/vertical transmission**
4. **Breast feeding**
5. **Blood splash on open wound/eyes**

2.2 What grade of infectivity does the blood result imply? [Marks 1]
High infectivity

2.3 What three measures would you recommend for this woman's newborn baby? [Marks 3]
1. **Active immunisation/hepatitis B vaccination**
2. **Passive immunisation/hepatitis B immunoglobin**
3. **Avoidance of breast feeding if possible**

2.4 How soon should the newborn baby be immunised?
[Marks 1]
Within 24 hours

2.5 Of those infected babies perinatally, what percentage will become chronic carriers? [Marks 1]
90%

3.1 Comment on the two trends shown. [Marks 2]
There is a fall in both absolute numbers of deaths and the rates of death per million maternities over the three triennia.

3.2 In 1991–1993, substandard care was identified in 80% of cases? How does this compare with previous triennia? [Marks 1]
No significant change

3.3 Two factors have consistently been identified as contributing to the substandard care. What are these? [Marks 2]
1. **Failure to take prompt action**
2. **Inadequate/late consultant involvement**

3.4 In 1991–1993, 11 deaths followed eclampsia. In none of these cases was magnesium sulphate used. How may this change and why? [Marks 2]
There will be a likely increase in the usage of magnesium sulphate following the findings of the collaborative eclampsia trial (1995)

3.5 Give three recommendations made at the end of the 1991–1993 report with regard to hypertensive disease in pregnancy. [Marks 3]
1. **SHO not to be given responsibility for executive decisions**
2. **Strict attention to fluid balance**
3. **Formation of a specialist team with a lead obstetrics consultant**
4. **Ergometrine/Syntometrine to be avoided unless there is severe postpartum haemorrhage**
5. **Improvement in standard and compliance rates of autopsy**

4.1 With regards to BP in pregnancy, what normally happens in the first trimester? [Marks 1]
BP drops

4.2 What happens in the second trimester normally? [Marks 1]
BP drops more significantly

4.3 What happens in the third trimester normally? [Marks 1]
BP returns to first trimester levels

4.4 What features are you concerned about with Mrs EF? Name two. [Marks 2]
   1. **BP has risen significantly at 32 weeks**
   2. **Proteinuria has developed**

4.5 What do you arrange now? Name three measures. [Marks 3]
   1. **MSU**
   2. **FBC and platelets**
   3. **Serum urate**
   4. **Refer to day assessment unit or recheck BP in 2 days**

4.6 In the latest maternal mortality report (1991–1993), where did hypertensive diseases rate among the commonest causes of direct deaths? [Marks 1]
Second

4.7 In deaths from hypertensive disease, what was the commonest cause? [Marks 1]
Adult respiratory distress syndrome

5.1 What is the first thing you do when you enter the room (apart from introducing yourself). [Marks 1]
Rub up a contraction

5.2 What two relevant questions do you ask the midwife? [Marks 2]
   1. **Has she had ergometrine/Syntocinon with the anterior shoulder?**
   2. **Was the placenta complete?**

5.3 What do you then do? Name five courses of action.
[Marks 5]
1. **Call senior help**
2. **IV line**
3. **Blood for cross match**
4. **FBC**
5. **Syntocinon/ergometrine**
6. **Clotting studies**

5.4 What is the most likely cause? [Marks 1]
Atonic uterus

5.5 You are unable to stop the bleeding. What measure do you take while awaiting senior help? [Marks 1]
Bimanual compression

STATION 6 ANSWERS **CIRCUIT C**

6.1 List five features that place her in a high risk category for pregnancy which would have been identified at the booking visit. [Marks 5]
1. **Primigravida**
2. **Smoker**
3. **Maternal weight > 100 kg**
4. **Unsupported/(single mother)**
5. **Unsure dates**

6.2 Comment on her 24 and 26 weeks' visits to her midwife. [Marks 1]
Persistent 2 + glycosuria

6.3 What investigation would you have arranged? [Marks 1]
Oral glucose tolerance test (GTT)

6.4 She is seen in the hospital antenatal clinic around 32 weeks. Comment on the abdominal findings. [Marks 1]
Clinically small for dates

6.5 What investigation would you arrange at this visit? [Marks 1]
USS for growth and liquor

6.6 At 38/40, Ms HP is delivered of a 2.1 kg baby boy by LSCS. Comment on this. [Marks 1]
Confirmed small for gestational age baby

7.1 What has happened? [Marks 1]

Partial breakdown of episiotomy repair

7.2 List four factors which may predispose to this complication. [Marks 4]
1. **Poor repair technique**
2. **Perineal wound haematoma**
3. **Perineal wound infection**
4. **Poor hygiene after repair**
5. **Undiagnosed third degree tear**
6. **Maternal diabetes**
7. **HIV infection**

7.3 In the absence of infection, how is this complication best managed? Specify two points. [Marks 2]
1. **Careful hygiene/surgical toilet**
2. **Allow healing by secondary intention/granulation**

7.4 List three simple measures which may improve symptoms. [Marks 3]
1. **Simple analgesia**
2. **Anti-inflammatory drugs**
3. **Stool softeners**
4. **Inflatable rubber ring (to sit on)**

8.1 What abnormality is shown? [Marks 1]
Shortened 4th metacarpal of the left hand

8.2 What is the most likely diagnosis? [Marks 1]
Turner's syndrome

8.3 If you analysed her chromosomes, what would they show? [Marks 1]
XO

8.4 What hormone test would you request? [Marks 1]
Follicle stimulating hormone (FSH)

8.5 What would her uterus look like? [Marks 1]
Rudimentary/hypoplastic

8.6 What would her gonads look like? [Marks 1]
Absent or streak ovaries

8.7 What hormonal replacement would you give her? [Marks 1]
Oestrogen and progestogens/COC pill/HRT

8.8 Name two conditions under which this woman could become pregnant. [Marks 2]
1. **If she was a Turner's mosaic**
2. **Oocyte donation**

8.9 Name one way this condition could have been detected during her mother's pregnancy. [Marks 2]
1. **USS**
2. **Amniocentesis**
3. **Chorionic villous sampling (CVS)**

STATION 9	ANSWERS	CIRCUIT C

9.1 What do you see? [Marks 1]
Tumour on the vulva

9.2 What is the most likely diagnosis? [Marks 1]
Vulva carcinoma

9.3 What is the most common histological diagnosis? [Marks 1]
Squamous carcinoma

9.4 Which nodes would this spread to? [Marks 1]
1. **Inguinal and femoral nodes**
2. **Deep pelvic nodes**

9.5 What is the treatment of choice? [Marks 2]
Radical vulvectomy and bilateral groin node dissection

9.6 What is the 5-year survival rate for node negative stage 1 cases? [Marks 1]
95%

9.7 Name three predisposing factors for this condition. [Marks 3]
1. **Chronic vulval irritation**
2. **Premalignant disease of vagina**
3. **Premalignant disease of cervix**

10.1 What abnormality does it show? [Marks 1]
Fibroid uterus

10.2 Name three symptoms she may have presented with?
[Marks 3]
1. **Abdominal distension**
2. **Infertility**
3. **Difficulty with micturition**
4. **Abdominal pain**
5. **Menorrhagia**

10.3 If she was to have this abnormality removed by a
conservative procedure, what intraoperative complications
may arise? Name two. [Marks 2]
1. **Haemorrhage**
2. **Damage to other organs, e.g. ureter, bladder, bowel**

10.4 What must a patient be warned about prior to this
operation? [Marks 1]
**A blood transfusion and/or hysterectomy may be
needed.**

10.5 If this woman had become pregnant prior to her operation,
name two complications that she may have had during the
pregnancy. [Marks 2]
1. **Abnormal lie**
2. **Urinary retention**
3. **Placental abruption/APH**

10.6 In what percentage of cases may this condition be
malignant? [Marks 1]
0.2%

11.1 What does the result suggest? [Marks 1]
Premalignant disease of the cervix/cervical precancer

11.2 What investigation is indicated? [Marks 2]
1. **Colposcopy**
2. **Colposcopic biopsy**

11.3 Name two solutions used to identify abnormal areas on the
cervix. [Marks 2]
1. **Acetic acid**
2. **Lugol's iodine/iodine**

11.4 The squamo-columnar junction is wholly visible and biopsy of a clearly defined abdominal area confirms CIN II. List three methods suitable for removing the abnormal area. [Marks 3]
1. **Cold coagulation**
2. **Diathermy ablation**
3. **Diathermy excision**
4. **Laser ablation**
5. **LLETZ**

11.5 If the extent of the abnormal area is not visible, which diagnostic procedure is indicated? [Marks 1]
1. **Knife cone biopsy**
2. **Large loop cone**
3. **Laser cone biopsy**

11.6 Given Mrs CD's menstrual history, what other surgical options should be considered? Name one. [Marks 1]
1. **Total abdominal hysterectomy**
2. **Vaginal hysterectomy**

STATION 12 ANSWERS	**CIRCUIT C**

12.1 What is this investigation called? [Marks 1]
Hysterosalpingogram

12.2 Describe the findings. Specify two features. [Marks 2]
1. **Normal outline of the uterine cavity**
2. **Dilated tubal lumen; no spillage**
3. **Bilateral hydrosalpinges**

12.3 What is the commonest microorganism leading to this picture? [Marks 1]
Chlamydia (trachomatis)

12.4 In the presence pf normal ovulation and a normal semen analysis in her partner, what are the two options for facilitating conception in this patient? [Marks 2]
1. **Tubal surgery/microsurgery/salpingostomy**
2. **In vitro fertilisation**

12.5 What is the usually quoted take-home baby rate following in vitro fertilisation in experienced hands? [Marks 1]
20–30%

12.6 List three important complications of IVF. [Marks 3]
1. **Ovarian hyperstimulation**
2. **Multiple pregnancy**
3. **Ectopic pregnancy**
4. **Miscarriage**
5. **Failed conception**
6. **Congenital malformation**

| STATION 13 | ANSWERS | CIRCUIT C |

13.1 List three investigations you would arrange during your speculum examination. [Marks 3]
1. **Cervical smear**
2. **Endocervical swab for chlamydia**
3. **High vaginal swab for microscopy culture and sensitivity**

13.2 Speculum examination reveals a florid ectropion. Which of her symptoms might this cause? Name two. [Marks 2]
1. **Discharge**
2. **Postcoital bleeding**
3. **Dyspareunia in the presence of cervicitis**

13.3 If the investigations performed in Question 13.1 were normal, how would you treat the ectropion? [Marks 1]
Cryocautery/cold coagulation/diathermy/laser

13.4 Name the structure shown in B. [Marks 1]
Hodge pessary

13.5 What is this used for? [Marks 2]
Reversible anteversion of a mobile retroverted uterus

13.6 Use of B results in the alleviation of symptoms. Which operation would you recommend? [Marks 1]
Ventrosuspension

| STATION 14 | ANSWERS | CIRCUIT C |

14.1 Look at the result shown. Name the investigation. [Marks 1]
Subtraction cystometry and uroflowmetry/urodynamic studies

14.2 Define a normal urinary flow rate for a woman. [Marks 1]
> 15 ml/s

14.3 What is the abnormality shown? [Marks 1]
Genuine stress incontinence

14.4 What simple measures may improve the patient's symptoms? Name two. [Marks 2]
1. **Weight loss**
2. **Stop smoking**
3. **Treat constipation**
4. **Pelvic floor exercises**
5. **Physiotherapy**
6. **Faradism**
7. **Vaginal cones**

14.5 List three surgical approaches to treat this condition, and provide an example of each. [Marks 3]
1. **Vaginal approach, e.g. anterior colporraphy/Pacey/Kelly repair**
2. **Abdominal approach, e.g. Burch colposuspension/Marshall–Marchetti–Krantz**
3. **Combined abdominovaginal approach, e.g. Stamey procedure**

14.6 Which operation has the highest documented success rate? [Marks 1]
Colposuspension

14.7 What is the usually quoted success rate in experienced hands? [Marks 1]
80–90%

STATION 15	ANSWERS	CIRCUIT C

15.1 Give three possible uterine causes of the pain. [Marks 3]
1. **Preterm labour**
2. **Abruption**
3. **Fibroid degeneration**
4. **Chorioamnionitis**

15.2 Give three possible non-uterine causes of the pain. [Marks 3]
1. **Urinary tract infection (UTI)**
2. **Constipation**
3. **Appendicitis**
4. **Ovarian cyst (accident)**
5. **Gastroenteritis**
6. **Inflammatory bowel disease**

15.3 What clinical signs would you look for on examination to help you make a diagnosis? [Marks 4]
1. **Pyrexia**
2. **Tachycardia/hypotension/shock**
3. **Uterus – soft or tense/contractions/tender**
4. **Vaginal examination – cervical change (effacing, dilation)/evidence of SROM/discharge**
5. **Abdominal – tenderness/guarding**
6. **Renal angle tenderness**

STATION 16 ANSWERS	**CIRCUIT C**

16.1 Define the term teratogen. [Marks 1]
A teratogen is a substance that causes structural or functional abnormality in a fetus exposed to that substance.

16.2 What is the approximate molecular weight of substances which readily cross the placenta? [Marks 1]
Molecular weight less than 1000

16.3 List the three phases of development of a conceptus and specify the precise timing in completed weeks post-conception. [Marks 6]
1. **Pre-embryonic phase: 0–2 weeks**
2. **Embryonic phase: 3–8 weeks**
3. **Fetal phase: 9 weeks to birth**

16.4 At which of these phases does exposure to a teratogen have the greatest potential to cause gross malformation? [Marks 1]
Embryonic phase

16.5 What criteria must be satisfied before prescribing a pregnant woman a known teratogen? [Marks 1]
The potential benefit(s) to the mother must outweigh or justify the risk to the fetus.

17.1 What is the incidence of spontaneous twins in the UK? [Marks 1]
1:80

17.2 This incidence is rising. Why? [Marks 1]
As a result of assisted conception/ovulation induction regimes

17.3 What percentage of twins are monozygotic? [Marks 1]
28–30%

17.4 Graphs 1 and 2 show serial ultrasound measurements of abdominal and head circumference in a monochorionic–diamniotic twin pregnancy. Describe three findings. [Marks 3]
   1. Twin 1 is growing normally along the 50th centile
   2. Twin 2 has a decreasing abdominal circumference
   3. Twin 2 has a normal head circumference (except head sparing/asymmetrical growth retardation)

17.5 Graph 3 shows serial amniotic fluid index measurements from the two sacs. Describe two findings. [Marks 2]
   1. Twin 1 has normal liquor
   2. Twin 2 has reduced liquor/oligohydramnios

17.6 What term is used to describe this sequence of events? [Marks 1]
   IUGR in twin 2

17.7 Umbilical arterial Doppler of twin 2 shows reversed end diastolic flow. What would you arrange? [Marks 1]
   1. Emergency lower segment caesarean section
   2. Fetal cord blood sample

18.1 Define preterm delivery. [Marks 1]
This is delivery occurring after 24 completed weeks of gestation but prior to 37 completed weeks of gestation.

18.2 What is the incidence of preterm delivery? [Marks 1]
Approximately 10% of all deliveries

18.3 List four risk factors for preterm delivery in Miss PL's history. [Marks 4]
1. **Age < 16 years**
2. **Cigarette smoking**
3. **Low socioeconomic class**
4. **Previous mid-trimester evacuation termination**

18.4 What examinations would you carry out to establish a diagnosis of preterm labour? Specify two. [Marks 2]
1. **Abdominal palpation (to assess intensity frequency and duration of contractions)**
2. **Serial cervical assessment (to assess change in effacement/consistency/dilatation of the cervix)**

18.5 In the presence of preterm labour, what would you administer to Miss PL to encourage fetal lung maturation? Specify preparation, dose, route of administration and frequency. [Marks 2]
Dexamethasone 12 mg intramuscularly (two doses separated by 12 hours), or betamethasone 12 mg intramuscularly (two doses separated by 12 hours)

STATION 19	ANSWERS	CIRCUIT C

19.1 What would you advise her about the rate of vertical transmission? [Marks 1]
11–30%

19.2 During the pregnancy, her CD4 count is <200 mm^3 on three occasions. What would you give her for prophylaxis against *Pneumocystis carinii* pneumonia (PCP)? [Marks 1]
Cotrimoxazole 960 mg daily on 3 days a week

19.3 She develops oral candidiasis. What would you give her? [Marks 1]
Nystatin oral suspension

19.4 This appears to be ineffective. What would you offer her? [Marks 1]
Fluconazole

19.5 Would you give her folic acid? Justify your answer. [Marks 1]
No. Folic acid may exacerbate infection with toxoplasmosis

19.6 What iron preparation would you give her? [Marks 1]
Ferrous sulphate

19.7 Does caesarean section offer any advantage with regard to vertical transmission? [Marks 1]
Yes. It probably decreases it by about 20%.

19.8 How long does it take for the baby to lose maternal antibody? [Marks 1]
Up to 18 months

19.9 What immunisations should the baby not be given? Name two. [Marks 1]
   1. **Live oral polio vaccine, as there is a theoretical risk of causing persistent infection in children or harm to HIV-infected family members**
   2. **BCG**

STATION 20 ANSWERS   **CIRCUIT C**

20.1 Describe the appearance of the uterine cavity. [Marks 1]
A central sac in the uterus (pseudosac)

20.2 Describe the finding to the left of the uterus. [Marks 1]
A true gestation sac with an identifiable fetus

20.3 Where is the answer to Question 20.2 likely to be located? [Marks 1]
In the left fallopian tube

20.4 Miss EP is haemodynamically stable with no signs of peritonism. State four different methods of treating her condition. [Marks 4]
   1. **Intravenous methothrexate**
   2. **Intratubal methothrexate guided by ultrasound**
   3. **Intratubal saline/methothrexate under laparoscopic control**
   4. **Laparoscopic salpingotomy/salpingectomy**
   5. **Laparotomy and salpingotomy/salpingectomy**

20.5 If a laparoscopic conservative procedure is performed, when would you expect Miss EP to be well enough to go home? [Marks 1]
Within 24 hours/the next day

20.6 How should she be followed up? [Marks 1]
**With serial serum BHCG quantitation separated by
48–72 hours**

20.7 What is currently the most common aetiological factor
associated with ectopic pregnancy? [Marks 1]
Pelvic inflammatory disease/chlamydia infection

CIRCUIT D

1.1 What eponym is given to this test?

1.2 Specify two features which would lead you to suspect an abnormal result.

1.3 Name the condition that this test is designed to detect?

1.4 How common is this condition?

1.5 What percentage of babies with an abnormal screening test result actually have the condition?

1.6 Is there a sex difference in incidence? Please specify.

1.7 Name an important obstetric risk factor.

1.8 If the screening test is positive, to whom should the baby be referred?

1.9 In the presence of a persistently abnormal result, what is the first line of treatment?

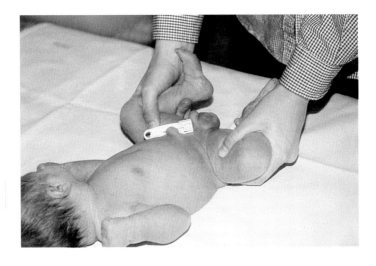

2.1   What object is seen?

2.2   What does this object do?

2.3   What other objects can be used? Name two.

2.4   What is this procedure called?

2.5   What is the failure rate of this procedure?

2.6   Name two points you would ensure the couple understood about the procedure.

2.7   Name two reasons for this procedure failing.

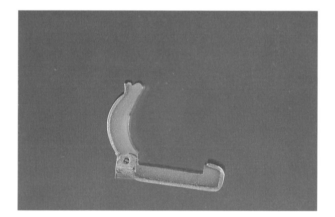

3.1 Describe what you see.

3.2 What is this syndrome called?

3.3 What is the most likely organism?

3.4 In the outpatients' department, what specimen would you take to detect this organism?

3.5 Name two antibiotics to which this organism is sensitive.

3.6 If a neonate is exposed to chlamydia, what may he/she develop?

3.7 If a male had this organism, name the clinical diagnosis.

3.8 What other organism may cause the above appearance?

3.9 What is the treatment?

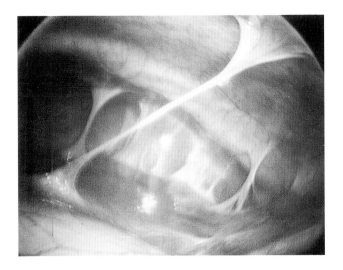

4.1 What do the letters NCEPOD stand for?

4.2 When was this regular enquiry launched?

4.3 Which deaths are included in the enquiry?

4.4 Who is the usual reporting clinician?

4.5 The table shown is taken from the 1991–1992 report where there was a special enquiry into deaths following hysterectomy (Dept of Health). In what proportion of cases that resulted in death was the consultant involved in the decision to operate?

4.6 How does this figure compare with that of the index cases?

4.7 In what proportion of the cases resulting in death was the decision for hysterectomy made by a junior trainee (SHO or registrar)?

4.8 How does this compare with the index group?

4.9 Please comment.

Grade of most senior surgeon consulted prior to hysterectomy		
Grade	**Deaths (65)**	**Index (468)**
SHO		1
Registrar	2	6
Senior registrar	3	17
Consultant	60	437
Staff grade		1
Not recorded		6
Adapted from NCEPOD report 1992, Department of Health		

A sample of urine is provided from a 32 week primigravida patient with BP 160/100 mmHg, with no past history of note. The urine is tested with BM stix.

5.1 What substance has been detected?

5.2 What is the concentration in grams per litre?

5.3 What other maternal investigations would you arrange? Name five.

5.4 What is your management?

5.5 Name the two most likely diagnoses.

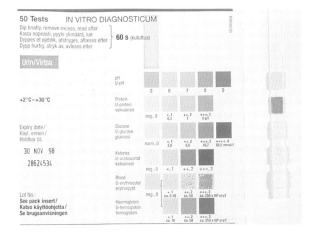

The specimen was produced from a postpartum hysterectomy. The woman had uterine inversion during the third stage.

6.1 What caused the uterine inversion? Name two problems.

6.2 How do you initially manage uterine inversion?

6.3 If your first manoeuvre fails, what do you do?

6.4 Why do you think this women had a hysterectomy?

6.5 Name three intraoperative complications that may occur during a postpartum hysterectomy.

6.6 Would the ovaries be removed at the time of operation?

6.7 Name one predisposing factor to the underlying pathology.

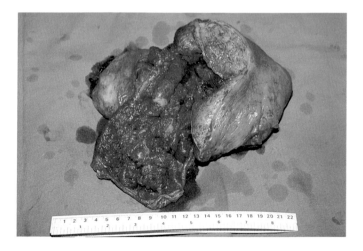

Mrs AS is a 22-year-old Nigerian woman in her first pregnancy. Her booking haemoglobin electrophoresis result is shown.

7.1 What haemoglobinopathy does Mrs AS have?

7.2 Who else should be tested?

7.3 If Mrs DF's partner also has the same haemoglobinopathy, what are the respective chances of the fetus being normal, having the same haemoglobinopathy as either parent or the overt disease?

7.4 What has been the usual method for prenatal diagnosis of haemoglobinopathy in the fetus? Specify the tissue sample and the test.

7.5 At what gestation is this usually performed?

7.6 State two other sources of DNA which allow earlier diagnosis of haemoglobinopathy.

Guy's Hospital	Surname	F
Department of Haematology	Forename	D
Date 27.10.97	Sex	F
	DOB	27.9.75
	Number	630927

Haemoglobin Electrophoresis
H6 A	65%
H6 S	30%
H6 F	3%

Mrs ST had a normal delivery of a baby boy 2 weeks ago. She has been breast feeding her son and has recently developed 'flu-like' symptoms. Her left breast has become swollen and painful, and on examination she has a temperature of 38.2°C but there is no sign of an upper respiratory tract infection. A photograph of her breasts is shown.

8.1   Describe the appearance of the left breast.

8.2   What is the diagnosis?

8.3   What is the usual infective organism?

8.4   How is this best treated? Give the name of the preparation, and the route, dose and frequency.

8.5   Specify two factors which may contribute to this clinical picture?

8.6   Mrs ST develops a purulent exudate from her left nipple. What should you advise? Name two features.

8.7   What further complication is she at risk from?

8.8   If this latter complication occurs, how should it be treated?

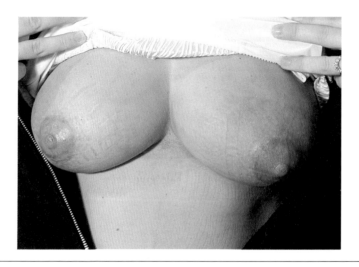

Mrs MA is a Caucasian woman in her second pregnancy. She has a 1-year-old girl and has not had a period for 13 weeks. She initially suffered with severe nausea but this subsequently resolved and she has been well for the last 4 weeks. During the last 48 hours, she has been experiencing a dark brown vaginal loss. A transvaginal ultrasound scan has been performed and a photograph of the findings is shown.

9.1 Describe the findings in the uterine cavity. Name two features.

9.2 What embryonic measurement is shown?

9.3 State the numerical value of the measurement and the corresponding gestational age.

9.4 During real-time scanning, the fetal heart is identified but is not seen beating. What is the diagnosis?

9.5 Which two haematological tests would you arrange?

9.6 Name the procedure that is indicated and the usual anaesthetic used.

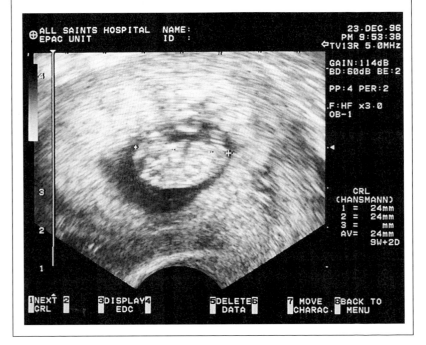

Mrs HF is 23 years old and in her second pregnancy. A blood result taken at 12 weeks by her midwife is shown.

10.1 What does the blood result show?

10.2 What proportion of the UK population have rhesus-negative blood?

10.3 In the presence of a rhesus-positive fetus, what condition may affect the fetus as a result of this level of anti-D antibody in the maternal serum?

10.4 Which immunoglobulin is responsible for the condition in the fetus?

10.5 What antigen does it bond to?

10.6 Where are these cells destroyed?

10.7 List four events in a pregnancy that may be associated with a significant fetomaternal haemorrhage.

Guy's Hospital **Department of Blood Transfusion**	Surname _____ F _____
	Forename _____ H _____
Date 10.10.97	Sex _____ F _____
	DOB _____ 11.11.93 _____
	Number _____ 731111 _____
Blood Group	A Rhesus Negative
Atypical Antibodies	Present
Specificity	Anti-D Antibodies
Quantitation	8 iu/ml

11.1 What is the illustrated instrument used for?

11.2 Name two important contraindications.

11.3 Where is transcutaneous electrical nerve stimulation (TENS) placed? Name two sites.

11.4 Name two side-effects of nitrous oxide.

11.5 What is the most serious maternal side-effect of pethidine?

11.6 Why should pethidine not be used in fulminating pre-eclampsia?

11.7 What nerve roots does the pudendal nerve arise from?

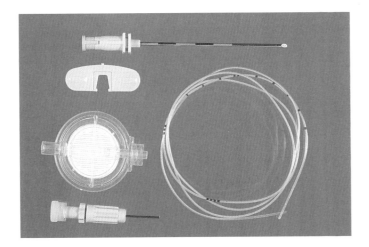

12.1 What is shown in this photograph?

12.2 Name four features that are normal.

12.3 If a fetus is distressed, what features would you expect? Name three.

12.4 In labour, how else can fetal well-being be assessed? Name two methods.

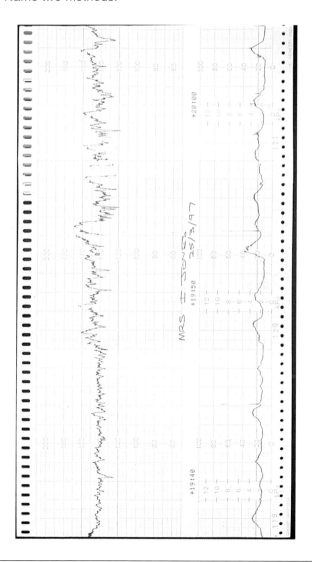

This baby is 2 days old and was 4.8 kg at birth.

13.1 What is the term used to describe this baby?

13.2 How may this have been detected antenatally. Name two methods.

13.3 What problem may have occurred in labour?

13.4 What problem may have occurred at delivery?

13.5 What problems may the baby develop neonatally? Name four.

13.6 Where should the baby be cared for during the first 24 hours?

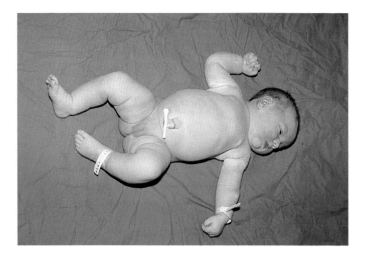

The specimen shown was obtained from a 66-year-old woman.

14.1 What is the most likely symptom that she may have presented with?

14.2 Name three risk factors for this condition?

14.3 What is the most likely histological diagnosis?

14.4 What is the premalignant phase histologically?

14.5 Where does it usually spread to? Name two sites.

14.6 What is the treatment for early stage disease?

14.7 What is the 5-year survival for stage 1 disease?

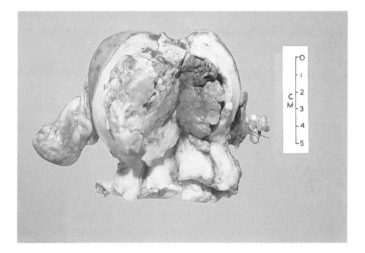

Miss TD is 17 years old and has had 11 weeks of amenorrhoea. For the last 3 weeks she has complained of nausea and vomiting and she has had heavy vaginal bleeding for 2 days.

15.1 An ultrasound has been performed. What does this show?

15.2 What does this appearance suggest?

15.3 What is the prevalence of this condition in the UK?

15.4 List two predisposing factors for this condition?

15.5 Which hormonal assay is useful in the management of this condition?

15.6 What is the treatment?

15.7 Histology confirms your diagnosis. How would you follow up Miss TD? Specify the test, where this should be performed, the frequency and the duration.

15.8 What is the usual method of treating chorion carcinoma?

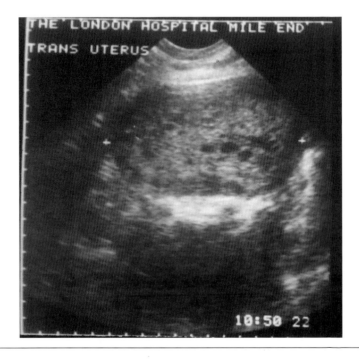

Mrs OT is 23 years old and presents to accident and emergency with a 6 hour history of constant right iliac fossa pain with intermittent gripping exacerbations. She has vomited on four occasions when the pain was at its worst. Her temperature is 37°C, there is guarding and rebound tenderness in the lower abdomen and she has marked tenderness in the right fornix. Her full blood count and transvaginal ultrasound report are shown.

16.1 What is the likely diagnosis?

16.2 List three important differential diagnoses.

16.3 What is the definitive investigation?

16.4 How soon should this investigation be performed? Explain why.

16.5 You confirm your diagnosis with your definitive investigation. Describe the principles of surgical management. Specify three.

Guy's Hospital
Department of Haematology

Date 12.12.97

Surname	T
Forename	O
Sex	F
DOB	12.11.74
Number	741112

Haemoglobin	12.5 g/dl
White cell count	17.6×10^9/l
Platelet count	199×10^{12}/l

Guy's Hospital
Department of Radiology

Date 1.5.98

Surname	T
Forename	O
Sex	F
DOB	12.11.74
Number	741112

Transvaginal ultrasound report

The uterus is anteverted and measures 12 × 5 cm.
A midline echo is seen.
The left ovary measures 3 × 2.8 × 4 cm.
A 7 cm cystic area of mixed echogenicity is seen on the right and appears to arise from the right ovary.
Free fluid is seen in the peritonal cavity.
Note: marked discomfort on introducing probe, particularly on the right.

This woman presented to the clinic complaining of regular heavy periods for 2 years. Her FBC is illustrated.

17.1 What is the normal blood loss per menstruation?

17.2 Name two terms to describe this woman's anaemia.

17.3 In the outpatient department, what would you do? Name three courses of action.

17.4 Name four medical treatments for menorrhagia.

Guy's Hospital **Department of Haematology**		Surname	P
		Forename	H
Date 2.9.97		Sex	F
		DOB	19.10.52
		Number	521019
Haemoglobin	7.6 g/dl		
White cell count	11.1×10^9/l		
Platelet count	247×10^{12}/l		
MCV	76 fl		
PCV	39%		
MCH	25 pg		
MCHC	27 g/dl		

The illustration shows a laparoscopic colposuspension being performed.

18.1 What is the medium used to distend the peritoneal cavity/cave of Retzius?

18.2 Name three complications that can occur on insertion of the trocar.

18.3 Name two safety measures performed prior to commencing laparoscopic surgery.

18.4 Name two advantages of a laparoscopic procedure over an open procedure for this patient.

18.5 What must the patient be prepared to accept when embarking upon any laparoscopic procedure?

18.6 If a patient complains of shoulder tip pain after a laparoscopy, what is the most likely cause?

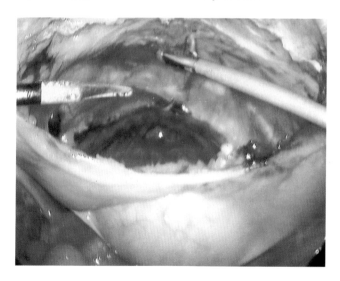

These laparoscopic views were obtained from a woman who presented with pelvic pain.

19.1 What is the diagnosis?

19.2 Name two signs you may have found on pelvic examination in the outpatient clinic?

19.3 Name three theories of the pathogenesis of this disease.

19.4 Name three medical treatments.

19.5 What is the incidence of this disease?

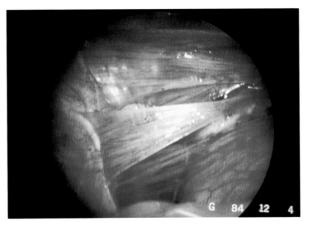

A

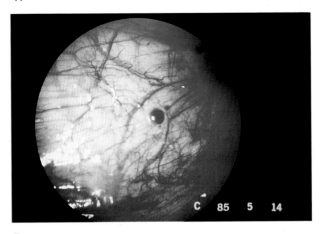

B

This woman presented with IMB.

20.1 What operation is being performed?

20.2 What can you see?

20.3 What management is indicated?

20.4 What other causes are there for IMB? Name three.

20.5 What media can be used to distend the cavity? Name two.

20.6 Is the histology likely to be benign or malignant?

20.7 How else might this problem have been diagnosed?

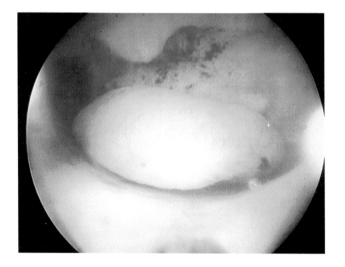

1.1 What eponym is given to this test? [Marks 1]
Ortolani's manoeuvre (test)

1.2 Specify two features which would lead you to suspect an abnormal result. [Marks 2]
1. Limited abduction of the hip
2. Clunk or click during active abduction

1.3 Name the condition that this test is designed to detect? [Marks 1]
Congenital dislocation of the hip

1.4 How common is this condition? [Marks 1]
1–2/1000 births

1.5 What percentage of babies with an abnormal screening test result actually have the condition? [Marks 1]
10–15%

1.6 Is there a sex difference in incidence? [Marks 1]
Yes; girls are more commonly affected than boys (6:1).

1.7 Name an important obstetric risk factor. [Marks 1]
Extended breech presentation

1.8 If the screening test is positive, to whom should the baby be referred? [Marks 1]
Orthopaedic surgeon/paediatric orthopaedic surgeon

1.9 In the presence of a persistently abnormal result, what is the first line of treatment? [Marks 1]
Abduction splint (Von Rosen splint)

2.1 What object is seen? [Marks 1]
Filschie clip

2.2 What does this object do? [Marks 1]
Occludes the tube

2.3 What other objects can be used? Name two. [Marks 2]
1. Hulka clip
2. Fallope ring

2.4 What is this procedure called? [Marks 1]
Sterilisation/laparoscopic sterilisation

2.5 What is the failure rate of this procedure? [Marks 1]
1 in 300 to 1 in 500

2.6 Name two points you would ensure the couple understood about the procedure. [Marks 2]
1. **Permanent procedure**
2. **Failure rate**

2.7 Name two reasons for this procedure failing.
1. **Clip applied to wrong structure**
2. **Incomplete application of clip to fallopian tube**

STATION 3 ANSWERS	**CIRCUIT D**

3.1 Describe what you see. [Marks 1]
Adhesions between the liver and the diaphragm.

3.2 What is this syndrome called? [Marks 1]
Fitz-Hugh Curtis syndrome

3.3 What is the most likely organism? [Marks 1]
Chlamydia

3.4 In the outpatients' department, what specimen would you take to detect this organism? [Marks 1]
Endocervical swab

3.5 Name two antibiotics to which this organism is sensitive. [Marks 2]
1. **Doxycycline**
2. **Erythromycin**

3.6 If a neonate is exposed to chlamydia, what may he/she develop? [Marks 1]
Conjunctivitis

3.7 If a male had this organism, name the clinical diagnosis. [Marks 1]
Non-specific urethritis (NSU)

3.8 What other organism may cause the above appearance? [Marks 1]
Gonorrhoea

3.9 What is the treatment? [Marks 1]
Penicillin

4.1 What do the letters NCEPOD stand for? [Marks 1]
The National Confidential Enquiry into Perioperative Deaths

4.2 When was this regular enquiry launched? [Marks 1]
1988

4.3 Which deaths are included in the enquiry? [Marks 2]
Deaths occurring in hospital within 30 days of a surgical procedure

4.4 Who is the usual reporting clinician? [Marks 1]
Consultant pathologist

4.5 The table shown is taken from the 1991–1992 report where there was a special enquiry into deaths following hysterectomy (Dept of Health). In what proportion of cases that resulted in death was the consultant involved in the decision to operate? [Marks 1]
92%

4.6 How does this figure compare with that of the index cases? [Marks 1]
Equivalent at 93%

4.7 In what proportion of the cases resulting in death was the decision for hysterectomy made by a junior trainee (SHO or registrar)? [Marks 1]
Two cases out of 65 (3%)

4.8 How does this compare with the index group? [Marks 1]
Seven out of 468 cases (1.5%)

4.9 Please comment. [Marks 1]
These figures are unacceptably high and a consultant or senior gynaecologist should be involved in all decisions for hysterectomy.

| STATION 5 | ANSWERS | CIRCUIT D |

5.1 What substance has been detected? [Marks 1]
Protein

5.2 What is the concentration in grams per litre? [Marks 1]
> 5 g/l

5.3 What other maternal investigations would you arrange? Name five. [Marks 5]
   1. **FBC and platelets**
   2. **U&E**
   3. **Urate**
   4. **24 hour urine**
   5. **Clotting studies**
   6. **Liver enzymes**

5.4 What is your management? [Marks 1]
   Admit to hospital

5.5 Name the two most likely diagnoses. [Marks 2]
   1. **Pre-eclampsia**
   2. **Renal disease**

STATION 6   ANSWERS   **CIRCUIT D**

6.1 What caused the uterine inversion? Name two problems. [Marks 2]
   1. **Pulling on the cord without suprapubic counter-traction to stop uterus inverting**
   2. **Morbid adherence of the placenta**

6.2 How do you initially manage uterine inversion? [Marks 1]
   Manually reverse inversion immediately

6.3 If your first manoeuvre fails, what do you do? [Marks 1]
   Hydrostatic method/O'Sullivan's method

6.4 Why do you think this women had a hysterectomy? [Marks 1]
   1. **Manual removal was unsuccessful and therefore laparotomy was performed, ending in hysterectomy**
   2. **Massive haemorrhage**

6.5 Name three intraoperative complications that may occur during a postpartum hysterectomy. [Marks 3]
   1. **Massive haemorrhage**
   2. **DIC**
   3. **Anaesthetic complications**
   4. **Damage to other structures, e.g. ureter, bladder**

6.6 Would the ovaries be removed at the time of operation? [Marks 1]
   No

6.7 Name one predisposing factor to the underlying pathology. [Marks 1]
1. **Implantation in the lower segment**
2. **Previous uterine scar**

| STATION 7 | ANSWERS | CIRCUIT D |

7.1 What haemoglobinopathy does Mrs AS have? [Marks 1]
Sickle cell trait

7.2 Who else should be tested? [Marks 1]
Mrs AS's partner

7.3 If Mrs DF's partner also has the same haemoglobinopathy, what are the respective chances of the fetus being normal, having the same haemoglobinopathy as either parent or the overt disease? [Marks 3]
1:4, 1:2, 1:4

7.4 What has been the usual method for prenatal diagnosis of haemoglobinopathy in the fetus? Specify the tissue sample and the test. [Marks 2]
Fetal blood sampling and analysis of globin synthesis genes

7.5 At what gestation is this usually performed? [Marks 1]
18–20 weeks

7.6 State two other sources of DNA which allow earlier diagnosis of haemoglobinopathy. [Marks 2]
1. **Amniotic fluid fibroblasts/amniocentesis**
2. **Chorion villus biopsy**

| STATION 8 | ANSWERS | CIRCUIT D |

8.1 Describe the appearance of the left breast. [Marks 1]
Engorged (swollen) with erythema

8.2 What is the diagnosis? [Marks 1]
Mastitis

8.3 What is the usual infective organism? [Marks 1]
Staphylococcus aureus

8.4 How is this best treated? Give the name of the preparation, and the route, dose and frequency. [Marks 1]
1. **Oral flucloxacillin 250 mg QDS**
2. **Oral erythromycin 250 mg QDS (in those allergic to penicillin)**

8.5 Specify two factors which may contribute to this clinical picture? [Marks 2]
1. **Incomplete emptying of breasts/milk stasis**
2. **Cracked or traumatised nipples**

8.6 Mrs ST develops a purulent exudate from her right nipple. What should you advise? [Marks 2]
1. **Discontinue feeding from the affected breast**
2. **Express manually from the affected breast**

8.7 What further complication is she at risk from? [Marks 1]
Breast abscess

8.8 If this latter complication occurs, how should it be treated? [Marks 1]
Incision and drainage

STATION 9	ANSWERS	CIRCUIT D

9.1 Describe the findings in the uterine cavity. Name two features. [Marks 2]
1. **Intrauterine gestation sac**
2. **Singleton fetus**

9.2 What embryonic measurement is shown? [Marks 1]
Crown rump length

9.3 State the numerical value of the measurement and the corresponding gestational age. [Marks 2]
24 mm (approximately equal to 9 weeks and 2 days of gestation)

9.4 During real-time scanning, the fetal heart is identified but is not seen beating. What is the diagnosis? [Marks 1]
Missed abortion

9.5 Which two haematological tests would you arrange? [Marks 2]
1. **Full blood count**
2. **Group and save**

9.6 Name the procedure that is indicated and the usual anaesthetic used. [Marks 2]
1. **Evacuation of retained products of conception**
2. **General anaesthetic**

10.1 What does the blood result show? [Marks 1]
Abnormally high level of anti-D antibody

10.2 What proportion of the UK population have rhesus-negative blood? [Marks 1]
17% (accept 15–20%)

10.3 In the presence of a rhesus-positive fetus, what condition may affect the fetus as a result of this level of anti-D antibody in the maternal serum? [Marks 1]
Haemolytic disease of the newborn/haemolytic anaemia/hydrops fetalis

10.4 Which immunoglobulin is responsible for the condition in the fetus? [Marks 1]
Maternal IgG

10.5 What antigen does it bond to? [Marks 1]
Fetal red cell D antigen

10.6 Where are these cells destroyed? [Marks 1]
Fetal spleen

10.7 List four events in a pregnancy that may be associated with a significant fetomaternal haemorrhage. [Marks 4]
1. **Miscarriage/bleeding in early pregnancy**
2. **Ectopic pregnancy**
3. **Amniocentesis/CVS/cordocentesis**
4. **APH**
5. **Delivery**
6. **Abdominal trauma**

11.1 What is the illustrated instrument used for? [Marks 1]
Epidural

11.2 Name two important contraindications. [Marks 2]
1. **Coagulopathy**
2. **Sepsis**
3. **Fixed output state**

11.3 Where is transcutaneous electrical nerve stimulation (TENS) placed? Name two sites. [Marks 2]
Over the posterior primary rami of T10–L1 and S2–S4

11.4 Name two side-effects of nitrous oxide. [Marks 2]
1. **Light-headedness**
2. **Nausea**

11.5 What is the most serious maternal side-effect of pethidine? [Marks 1]
Delaying gastric emptying

11.6 Why should pethidine not be used in fulminating pre-eclampsia? [Marks 1]
Because the major metabolite has convulsant properties

11.7 What nerve roots does the pudendal nerve arise from? [Marks 1]
S2, S3, S4

STATION 12	ANSWERS	CIRCUIT D

12.1 What is shown in this photograph? [Marks 1]
A cardiotocograph

12.2 Name four features that are normal. [Marks 4]
1. **Fetal heart rate of 140/min**
2. **Good variability of > 15 beats/min**
3. **Accelerations**
4. **Fetal movement**

12.3 If a fetus is distressed, what features would you expect? Name three. [Marks 3]
1. **Decelerations**
2. **Tachycardia**
3. **Bradycardia**
4. **Loss of variability**

12.4 In labour, how else can fetal well-being be assessed? Name two methods. [Marks 2]
1. **Liquor colour**
2. **Fetal blood sample**
3. **Umblical artery Doppler studies**

| STATION 13 | ANSWERS | CIRCUIT D |

13.1 What is the term used to describe this baby? [Marks 1]
Macrosomia

13.2 How may this have been detected antenatally. Name two methods. [Marks 2]
1. **Measuring symphysiofundal height**
2. **USS measurements**

13.3 What problem may have occurred in labour? [Marks 1]
Failure to progress

13.4 What problem may have occurred at delivery? [Marks 1]
Shoulder dystocia

13.5 What problems may the baby develop neonatally? Name four. [Marks 4]
1. **Hypoglycaemia**
2. **Hyperbilirubinaemia**
3. **Hypocalcaemia**
4. **Respiratory distress syndrome**
5. **Fitting/convulsions**

13.6 Where should the baby be cared for during the first 24 hours? [Marks 1]
In the special care baby unit

| STATION 14 | ANSWERS | CIRCUIT D |

14.1 What is the most likely symptom that she may have presented with? [Marks 1]
Postmenopausal bleeding

14.2 Name three risk factors for this condition? [Marks 3]
1. **Obesity**
2. **Polycystic ovarian syndrome (PCOS)**
3. **Nulliparity**
4. **Late menopause**
5. **Diabetes mellitus**
6. **Unopposed oestrogen therapy**

14.3 What is the most likely histological diagnosis? [Marks 1]
Adenocarcinoma

14.4 What is the premalignant phase histologically? [Marks 1]
Endometrial hyperplasia with atypia

14.5 Where does it usually spread to? Name two sites. [Marks 2]
1. **Myometrium**
2. **Pelvic lymph nodes**
3. **Para-aortic nodes**

14.6 What is the treatment for early stage disease? [Marks 1]
Total abdominal hysterectomy and bilateral salpingo-oopherectomy

14.7 What is the 5-year survival for stage 1 disease? [Marks 1]
75% (70–80%)

STATION 15	ANSWERS	CIRCUIT D

15.1 An ultrasound has been performed. What does this show? [Marks 1]
The appearance of vesicles

15.2 What does this appearance suggest? [Marks 1]
Hydatidiform mole

15.3 What is the prevalence of this condition in the UK? [Marks 1]
Approximately 1 in 1000 pregnancies

15.4 List two predisposing factors for this condition? [Marks 2]
1. **Extremes of reproductive age (<15 or >45 years)**
2. **South-east Asian origin**
3. **Blood groups AB or B**

15.5 Which hormonal assay is useful in the management of this condition? [Marks 1]
Human chorionic gonadotrophin (urine or serum)

15.6 What is the treatment? [Marks 1]
Suction evacuation of the uterus

15.7 Histology confirms your diagnosis. How would you follow up Miss TD? Specify the test, where this should be performed, the frequency and the duration. [Marks 2]
Urinary BHCG sent to a supraregional centre at fortnightly intervals for 6 months to 2 years

15.8 What is the usual method of treating chorion carcinoma? [Marks 1]
Chemotherapy/methotrexate

| STATION 16 | ANSWERS | CIRCUIT D |

16.1 What is the likely diagnosis? [Marks 1]
Ovarian torsion

16.2 List three important differential diagnoses. [Marks 3]
1. **Ectopic pregnancy**
2. **Ovarian cyst haemorrhage (rupture)**
3. **Appendicitis/PID**

16.3 What is the definitive investigation? [Marks 1]
Laparoscopy

16.4 How soon should this investigation be performed? Explain why. [Marks 2]
Immediately. Delay will lead to ovarian necrosis/irreversible damage.

16.5 You confirm your diagnosis with your definitive investigation. Describe the principles of surgical management? Specify three. [Marks 3]
1. **Untwist the ovarian pedicle**
2. **If the ovarian tissue looks viable, perform an ovarian cystectomy and conserve the ovary**
3. **If the ovary looks non-viable, remove the ovary**

| STATION 17 | ANSWERS | CIRCUIT D |

17.1 What is the normal blood loss per menstruation? [Marks 1]
Less than 80 ml

17.2 Name two terms to describe this woman's anaemia. [Marks 1]
1. **Microcytic**
2. **Hypochromic**

17.3 In the outpatient department, what would you do? Name three courses of action. [Marks 3]
1. **History**
2. **Pelvic examination**
3. **Endometrial biopsy/hysteroscopy**
4. **Smear if needed**
5. **Transvaginal ultrasound (TVS)**

17.4 Name four medical treatments for menorrhagia. [Marks 4]
1. **Danazol**
2. **NSAID/mefenamic acid**
3. **COC pill**
4. **Antifibrinolytics**
5. **Progestogens**
6. **Progestogen-containing IUCD**
7. **LHRH analogues**

18.1 What is the medium used to distend the peritoneal cavity/cave of Retzius? [Marks 1]
CO_2

18.2 Name three complications that can occur on insertion of the trocar. [Marks 3]
1. **Haemorrhage (inferior epigastric, iliac vessel)**
2. **Perforation of a viscus (bowel, baldder)**
3. **Failure to enter peritoneal cavity**

18.3 Name two safety measures performed prior to commencing laparoscopic surgery. [Marks 2]
1. **Diathermy pad on patient**
2. **Empty bladder**
3. **Check gas flow**
4. **Check equipment**

18.4 Name two advantages of a laparoscopic procedure over an open procedure for this patient. [Marks 2]
1. **Shorter hospital stay**
2. **Back to work quicker/back to normal activity**
3. **Better cosmesis**

18.5 What must the patient be prepared to accept when embarking upon any laparoscopic procedure? [Marks 1]
That a laparotomy may be needed

18.6 If a patient complains of shoulder tip pain after a laparoscopy, what is the most likely cause? [Marks 1]
CO_2 or blood irritating the diaphragm and causing referred pain to the shoulder tip

19.1 What is the diagnosis? [Marks 1]
Endometriosis

19.2 Name two signs you may have found on pelvic examination in the outpatient clinic? [Marks 2]
1. **A fixed retroverted uterus**
2. **Tender uterosacral ligaments with nodules**

19.3 Name three theories of the pathogenesis of this disease. [Marks 3]
1. **Coelomic metaplasia**
2. **Retrograde menstruation**
3. **Lymphatic/vascular spread**
4. **Immunological reaction**

19.4 Name three medical treatments. [Marks 3]
1. **Continuous COC pill**
2. **Danazol**
3. **GnRH analogues**
4. **Progestogens (high dose)**
5. **Gestrinone**

19.5 What is the incidence of this disease? [Marks 1]
10–40%

20.1 What operation is being performed? [Marks 1]
Hysteroscopy

20.2 What can you see? [Marks 1]
Endometrial polyp

20.3 What management is indicated? [Marks 1]
Removal of the polyp

20.4 What other causes are there for IMB? Name three. [Marks 3]
1. **Cervical polyp/cervical abnormality/cervical carcinoma**
2. **Endometrial hyperplasia**
3. **Endometrial carcinoma**
4. **Hormone therapy**
5. **Submucous fibroid**

20.5 What media can be used to distend the cavity? Name two.
[Marks 2]

1. **Normal saline**
2. **Glycine**
3. **CO_2**

20.6 Is the histology likely to be benign or malignant? [Marks 1]
Benign

20.7 How else might this problem have been diagnosed?
[Marks 1]
Transvaginal scan

COMMUNICATION AND STRUCTURED ORAL STATIONS

As this is a textbook rather than a live interactive situation, the demonstration of clinical and communication skills and structured oral stations is limited. The following examples will give you some idea as to what to expect. Prior to a communication station or structured oral station, there may be a rest station where information will be given to you for the actual communication/structured oral station. This will give you time to prepare for the encounter.

Remember that at the communication stations, communication is being assessed and knowledge is often secondary. The purpose of these stations is to assess your ability to communicate with the patients, so you must always treat them as individuals and be considerate. You want to convey to the examiner that you are a kind, compassionate and discerning clinician. As soon as you arrive at this station introduce yourself to the patient or the role-player. Remember that some patients are excellent historians and some are not. The role-player may have been briefed not to communicate well and therefore the station is assessing your skill to extract information. If there is a role-player at the station, she will have been briefed to give the same scenario to each candidate. The marking system will not be given to you and be aware that the role-player or patient may be awarding some marks.

With regard to structured orals, this scenario will involve yourself and the examiner. In some cases, the examiner may be role-playing, e.g. as a general practitioner, or may merely be asking you questions. There should be a logical flow to the structured oral. Whatever answer you give, the examiner may be instructed to present the contrary view. The following are examples of communication stations and structured orals.

Previous rest station – instructions to candidate

At the next station you will meet Mrs RT. She is a 34-year-old primigravida and she is currently at 37 weeks gestation. You need to check her BP, examine her abdomen and check for oedema.

Marking scheme	Marks
1. Introduction	1
2. Taking BP correctly (positioning etc.) and getting the correct BP	1
3. Observing the abdomen and detecting the laparoscopy scar	1
4. Measuring symphysiofundal height	1
5. Assessing presentation	1
6. Determining engagement of the head	1
7. Determining lie	1
8. Testing for oedema adequately	1

Marks from patient

1. Rapport	1
2. Not hurting patient during examination	1

Instructions to role-player
You have had pelvic pain premenstrually for 3 years. One year ago when you were in the States you had a laparoscopy and were told you had endometriosis. You did not attend for follow-up. Now you have come to see your GP/gynaecologist for an explanation about the disease and what treatments are available. Embarrassingly, you have recently noticed pain with intercourse and you suspect this may be related to endometriosis. You want to discuss endometriosis with the GP/gynaecologist and would like to bring up the problem with intercourse if he/she makes you feel comfortable enough.

Instructions to candidate
Your next patient has just booked under your care and has come for her first consultation.

Marking scheme	**Marks**
1. Introduction	1
2. Good rapport	1
3. Explaining the disease in easy terms	1
4. Being sympathetic	1
5. Explaining the options coherently	1
6. Extracting embarrassing problem	1

Marks from role-player

1. Felt confidence in candidate	1
2. Candidate gave good explanations	1
3. Would like to see him/her again	1
4. Candidate allowed role-player to choose between treatment options	1

Rest station – instructions to candidate
You are the SHO on call and you are about to take a phone call from a GP. When you arrive at the next station, pick up the telephone and speak to the GP.

Information to GP/examiner
You are a medical registrar and you know very little about gynaecology. You are doing a GP locum and a woman has arrived in your surgery with a history of unprotected intercourse 18 hours ago. You have no idea what to do, so rather embarrassingly you have rung the SHO on call in gynaecology. You want to find out what to do, when to do it and what the follow-up should be. You have heard that this certain SHO is rather arrogant so you are slightly on the defensive.

Marking scheme   **Marks**

1. Introduction	1
2. Fnding out what the problem is	1
3. Finding out when intercourse occurred	1
4. Being sympathetic to the GP's lack of knowledge regarding postcoital contraception	1
5. Clearly describing how to take the appropriate tablets	1
6. Discussing insertion IUCD	1
7. Checking that the GP has understood	1
8. Was the SHO overall easy to understand?	1
9. Was it obvious that the SHO knew what he was talking about?	1
10. Would you be happy to call this SHO about a problem again?	1

Information to candidate

You are the SHO on call. You receive a call from a local GP. He has been to see a 41-year-old nulliparous woman who has a 12 month history of very heavy irregular periods and on this occasion she is soaking a pad every 30 minutes and this has been occurring for 8 hours. He has telephoned you and wants you to admit the patient, but you feel you can handle it by giving telephone advice.

Instructions to local GP

Scenario as above. You want her admitted.

Marking scheme	Marks
1. SHO introducing himself on telephone	1
2. Being sympathetic to the GP's problem (woman distressed as bleeding at home)	1
3. Firmly refusing admission	1
4. Giving advice to stop bleeding – high dose progestogens	1
5. Advising the GP to check haemoglobin	1
6. Advising the GP to give iron	1
7. Arranging outpatient appointment	1
8. Reassuring the GP	1
9. Indicating what will happen in OP	1
10. Telling the GP to call back if he has further concerns	1

Information to candidate

A midwife has just seen Mrs RT at home. She is 39 weeks pregnant and complains of reduced fetal movements. The midwife has arranged a CTG which is shown to you as illustrated. Ask the midwife about any other information you think may be relevant and advise her regarding further management.

Information to midwife

Mrs RT is a 22-year-old primigravida at 39 weeks gestation. She is a healthy non-smoker and her antenatal course has been completely uneventful so far. Today she says the baby is not moving as much. Her blood pressure is 110/80 mmHg with no proteinuria and the baby appears clinically to be well grown with adequate liquor. You are not convinced that the CTG is abnormal enough to warrant intervention but have come to ask the doctor's opinion.

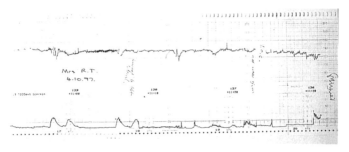

Marking scheme	**Marks**
1. Courteous and polite approach	1
2. Listening to the midwife	1
3. Obtaining other relevant history	1
4. Explaining that the CTG is abnormal and that the fetus should be delivered	1
5. Avoiding confrontational exchange	1
6. Giving clear instructions without appearing condescending	1
7. Asking the midwife if she has questions	1
8. Following verbal and non-verbal clues	1

Marks from midwife

| |
--- | ---
1. Confidence in the candidate's advice | 1
2. Candidate was not antagonistic | 1

Information to candidate

A community midwife comes to see you. She has seen Mrs EC, a 23-year-old primigravida at 32 weeks gestation, at home. Her booking blood pressure at 12 weeks was 110/60 mmHg and today it was 140/90 mmHg with + proteinuria. She asks your advice regarding further management.

Information to midwife

You have been to see Mrs EC at home. She is a 23-year-old healthy, non-smoking primigravida. She is 32 weeks pregnant with occasional headaches and she has noticed swelling of the fingers over the last 2 weeks. On examination, her blood pressure is 140/90 mmHg with + proteinuria. Abdominal examination reveals s sypmphysiofundal height of 26 cm, the presentation is cephalic and the fetus is active. You would like to manage the patient at home if possible.

Marking scheme

	Marks
1. Courteous and polite approach	1
2. Listening to the midwife	1
3. Obtaining other relevant information	1
4. Reassuring the midwife that the patient can be managed as an outpatient	1
5. Giving clear instructions regarding which investigations should be arranged	1
6. Giving clear instructions regarding indications for admission	1
7. Asking the midwife if she has any questions	1
8. Following verbal and non-verbal clues	1

Marks from midwife

1. Confidence in the candidate's advice	1
2. Rapport with the candidate	1

Information to candidate

Mrs AD is 43 years old and presents to your antenatal clinic at 10 weeks gestation in her second pregnancy. Her first pregnancy 2 years ago ended in miscarriage at 9 weeks. Her midwife has sent her to you to discuss antenatal diagnosis of congenital abnormalities. Counsel her regarding indications for antenatal tests and which tests are available.

Information to role-player

You are a very anxious 43-year-old and are worried about another miscarriage. You want as little interference with the pregnancy as possible and even if your baby had a congenital abnormality you would want to keep your baby. You are convinced that you will be forced to have an amniocentesis which will put your pregnancy at risk. During the consultation, ask these two specific questions:

- *Do I have to have an amniocentesis?*
- *Can't you see if the baby is alright on scan?*

Marking scheme   Marks

1. Introduction	1
2. Putting the patient at ease	1
3. Appropriate 'eye' contact	1
4. Listening to the patient	1
5. Extracting appropriate information	1
— wants little interference	
— would not terminate fetus	
6. Asking the patient if she has any questions	1
7. Reassuring that amniocentesis is not compulsory	1
8. Explaining that USS will pick up gross abnormalities but that chromosomal anomalies may be missed	1

Marks from role-player

1. Confidence in the candidate	1
2. Rapport	1

Information to candidate

Mrs TO is 29 years old and has a 7-year-old son from her previous marriage. She and her current partner have been trying to conceive for 2 1/2 years without success. Take a history from Mrs TO and explain the initial tests you are going to arrange – hormone profile and semen analysis.

Information to role-player

You are very anxious about not being able to have a baby. You stopped taking combined oral contraception 3 years ago and since then your periods have become very infrequent. In the last 6 months you have noticed a white discharge from the nipples. Do not offer this information unless specifically asked.

Your last menstrual period was 6 months ago. Your current partner is 26 and has two children from a previous marriage.

Marking scheme	**Marks**
1. Introduction	1
2. Putting the patient at ease	1
3. Appropriate 'eye' contact	1
4. Listening to the patient	1
5. Extracting appropriate information (amenorrhoea, galactorrhoea)	1
6. Explaining hormone profile	1
7. Explaining semen analysis	1
8. Asking if the patient has any questions	1

Marks from role-player	
1. Confidence in the candidate	1
2. Rapport	1

1.1 The examiner has three pairs of forceps in front of him/her, as shown in the photograph. Name the three forceps illustrated from top to bottom.

1.2 The examiner describes the following scenario: 'A woman has been pushing in the second stage for 2 hours and is exhausted; there is no head palpable abdominally and the head is at station +2, direct occipito-anterior.' Which forceps would you use?

1.3 The examiner says, 'Having decided to deliver by forceps, what type of analgesia could you use? Name two.

1.4 Before applying the forceps, what other requirements must you ensure have been met? Name two.

1.5 The examiner picks up the middle and lower forceps and asks you to name two differences between them.

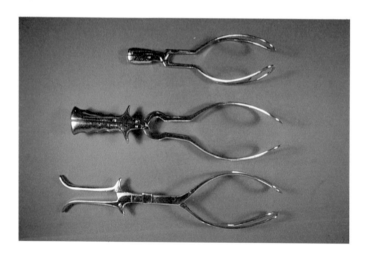

Rest station
Read the histology report below. The examiner at the next station will ask you some questions about it.

2.1 What procedure has been performed?

2.2 Describe the procedure.

2.3 The procedure was performed in colposcopy clinic. What anaesthetic would you have used?

2.4 Describe how you would carry out this procedure and what you would use.

2.5 Name two late complications of this procedure.

2.6 What further treatment would you suggest? Name two aspects.

Histology Report
Specimen measures 2.8 × 2.4 × 1.6 cm
The whole specimen has been processed. At the squamocolumnar junction there is extensive full-thickness cervical intraepithelial neoplasia III. The lesion appears to extend to the endocervical margins of excision, although this is difficult to determine as there is diathermy damage. There is no evidence of invasion.

Summary
CIN III, which may be incompletely excised. No evidence of invasion.

3.1 Describe the components shown in the box.

3.2 What is the appliance shown?

3.3 In general terms, after what type of surgical procedure is this appliance usually used?

3.4 What is the commonest complication of inserting such an appliance?

3.5 If this is suspected, what investigation is indicated?

3.6 If this complication is confirmed, which two measures should you aim to undertake?

Note: In the live situation, this question could involve you demonstrating catheter insertion on a pelvic model.

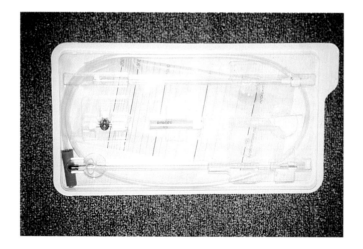

You are provided with a model of a fetal skull and female pelvis.

4.1 Demonstrate and describe the mechanism of normal labour.

4.2 Demonstrate:
1. **Deep transverse arrest**
2. **Occipitoposterior position**
3. **Brow presentation**
4. **Face presentation**

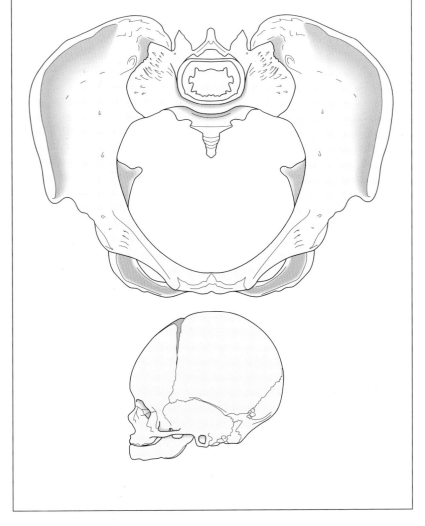

1.1 The examiner has three pairs of forceps in front of him/her, as shown in the photograph. Name the three forceps illustrated from top to bottom. [Marks 3]
1. **Wrigley's**
2. **Neville–Barnes/Anderson's/Simpson's**
3. **Kielland's**

1.2 The examiner describes the following scenario: 'A woman has been pushing in the second stage for 2 hours and is exhausted; there is no head palpable abdominally and the head is at station +2, direct occipito-anterior.' Which forceps would you use? [Marks 1]
Neville–Barnes (the middle one)

1.3 The examiner says, 'Having decided to deliver by forceps, what type of analgesia could you use? Name two.
[Marks 2]
1. **Epidural**
2. **Spinal**
3. **Pudendal**

1.4 Before applying the forceps, what other requirements must you ensure have been met? Name two. [Marks 2]
1. **Full dilatation of the cervix**
2. **Empty bladder**

1.5 The examiner picks up the middle and lower forceps and asks you to name two differences between them. [Marks 2]
1. **The lower one has a sliding lock**
2. **The middle one has both a cephalic and a pelvic curve, and the lower one has no pelvic curve**

2.1 What procedure has been performed? [Marks 1]
Large loop excision of the transformation zone (LLETZ)/laser cone/diathermy loop excision (DLE)

2.2 Describe the procedure. [Marks 2]
The diathermy loop is passed into the cervix and from right to left or from left to right and is then brought out. The specimen resembles a cone.

2.3 The procedure was performed in colposcopy clinic. What anaesthetic would you have used? [Marks 1]
Paracervical block

2.4 Describe how you would carry out this procedure and what you would use. [Marks 2]
Infiltrate at 3, 6, 9, 12 o'clock with an adrenalin-containing local anaesthetic

2.5 Name two late complications of this procedure. [Marks 2]
1. **Infertility**
2. **Cervical stenosis**
3. **Cervical incompetence**

2.6 What further treatment would you suggest? Name two aspects. [Marks 2]
1. **Follow-up smears**
2. **Repeat diathermy loop excision/cone biopsy**
3. **Hysterectomy**

STRUCTURED ORAL 3 ANSWERS

3.1 Describe the components shown in the box. Name four. [Marks 4]
1. **Three-way tap**
2. **Catheter connector**
3. **Catheter**
4. **Catheter bag**

3.2 What is the appliance shown? [Marks 1]
A suprapubic catheter (SPC)

3.3 In general terms, after what type of surgical procedure is this appliance usually used? [Marks 1]
Surgery to stabilise bladder neck/surgery for genuine stress incontinence

3.4 What is the commonest complication of inserting such an appliance? [Marks 1]
Urinary tract infection

3.5 If this is suspected, what investigation is indicated? [Marks 1]
CSU for microscopy/culture and sensitivity

OSCEs IN OBSTETRICS AND GYNAECOLOGY

3.6 If this complication is confirmed, which two measures should you aim to undertake? [Marks 2]
1. **Remove SPC as soon as practicable**
2. **Treat with appropriate antibiotics**

STRUCTURED ORAL 4	ANSWERS

4.1 Demonstrate and describe the mechanism of normal labour. [Marks 10]
One mark each is given for:
1. **Engagement**
2. **Flexion**
3. **Internal rotation**
4. **Descent**
5. **Extension**
6. **Restitution**

One mark each is given for demonstrating and describing:
1. **Deep transverse arrest**
2. **Occipitoposterior position**
3. **Brow presentation**
4. **Face presentation**